You Know Where It Hurts.
Now You Know Where to F̶ i̶ n̶ d̶ a̶ S̶ o̶ l̶ u̶ t̶ i̶ o̶ n̶.

Inside, discover:

• Detailed descriptions of specific ̶ p̶ a̶ i̶ n̶ s̶ i̶ n̶ parts of the body—such as an acute ̶ p̶ a̶ i̶ n̶ o̶ r̶ a burning sensation on the soles of your feet, a dull ache in your shoulder, a walnut-sized lump in your thigh—and exactly what those symptoms are telling you.

• The nature of your condition, what may have caused it, and how to prevent it from happening again.

• Notes on treatment and rehab, including suggestions about whether to apply ice or heat and the dangers of doing too much or too little.

• Whether to play through the pain or wait before getting back into the action—with strengthening exercises that can hasten the healing process.

◆

"Having benefited from Ben Gelfand's extraordinary expertise during the recovery of two knee surgeries (while performing the leads in two Broadway musicals), I can say without qualification the stuff in this book works! It's terrific!"

—Boyd Gaines

"If health is the key to happiness, then this book should have a generation of athletes jumping for joy."

—MVP Mike Richter,
all-star goaltender, New York Rangers

"A wonderful resource for the over-thirty athlete. I was quite impressed . . . the format is wonderful . . . I highly recommend RETURN TO GLORY DAYS."

—Barton Nisonson, M.D.,
team physician, New York Rangers

"The information here will prove a valuable asset to the older athlete. It's concise, accurate, and easy to read."

—Christina M. Morganti, M.D.,
sports medicine specialist

THE
RETURN
TO
GLORY DAYS

◆

Morton Dean

AND

Benjamin Gelfand, P.T.

POCKET BOOKS
New York   London   Toronto   Sydney   Tokyo   Singapore

ACKNOWLEDGMENTS

Benjamin Gelfand would like to thank Dr. James Nicholas, Dr. Stephen Nicholas, Dr. Bart Nisonson, and all his colleagues at the Nicholas Institute of Sports Medicine for their professionalism. Also thanks to his brother, Dr. Jeffrey Gelfand, for his help, and to his family for their love and support.

Morton Dean would like to thank Dr. James Nicholas and Ben Gelfand, his co-author, who have made the Glory Days games possible. Also thanks to our agent, Mitch Douglas at ICM, and to Paul McCarthy and Dan Slater at Pocket Books.

CONTENTS

Part Four

STRETCHES AND
STRENGTHENING EXERCISES   185

FOREWORD

by
JAMES A. NICHOLAS, MD
Founder of the Nicholas Institute of Sports Medicine and Athletic Trauma (NISMAT)

The importance of being physically active as long as one lives is widely accepted as an essential factor contributing to an improved quality of life. The human body, however, responds differently to an energetic athletic workout at different stages of life, even when one acquires basic fitness. Somewhere in the thirties, accumulated wear and tear, less time to stay fit, and the difficulty in staying motivated, all interact to increase many of our aches and pains.

This book provides a concise, winning way to help amateur athletes over thirty respond quickly to the "911 calls" they receive from their bodies. *The Return to Glory Days* does not speak in archaic terms or mystifying language. The book's outlines are straightforward, which makes the information easily accessible and appealing.

The authors should also be commended for recognizing and promoting an understanding of the theory of *linkage*, which is part of every aspect of fitness as well as injury. Overuse of the attachment sites between bones, ligaments, tendons, and muscles produces many subtle injuries that lead to the most common complaints resulting from athletic performance. These injuries can occur even at low levels of exercise intensity. We have learned from decades of dealing with highly skilled athletes that injury to one part of the body may affect another part of the body (hence the term "linkage"). When this principle is not recognized, the injury may produce weakness, instability, fatigue, or even additional problems at a later date. This book provides excellent explanations and insightful examples of how the principles of linkage can be applied to both the treatment of and the recovery from sports-related injuries.

Of course, the reader should realize that if there is a complicated type of unexplainable disability, or pain from a severe, more involved injury, he or she should consult with an orthopedic sports medicine specialist for an examination of the musculoskeletal system.

From reading this book, you will be able to accurately understand and properly address some of the more common and often ignored conditions of wear and tear that lead to more severe injuries, and less enjoyment, while playing sports. Equally important, this book will serve to motivate all to stay fit, pay attention to aches and pains, and learn what must be done in order to monitor and care for sports-related injuries.

Part One

INTRODUCTION

ACHES, PAINS, PULLS, AND STRAINS: HOW TO TREAT THEM AND HOW TO PREVENT THEM

If you're an active, over-thirty jock—man or woman—who has limped home, your psyche contorted by disappointment, your heart filled with despair about an ache or pain, wondering when you can get back into action, this book will become your constant companion and first point of reference.

Yes, there are other books about injuries and pain. And there are many books about exercising and getting into shape. But none is as specific, easy to read, or geared to your age group as this one.

Why does this book concentrate on age thirty and beyond? It has been firmly established that thirty is a departure point, when the body is in the process of important change and is becoming more susceptible to physical breakdowns caused by exercise and athletic competition. It's when the body begins to show signs of decreased flexibility and conditioning, weakening muscles, increased body fat, arthritis, and brittle bones. And for those reasons, among others, it's when the body begins to react differently to injuries, making recovery more difficult and reinjury more likely.

You'll find solace in the simplicity of *The Return to Glory Days*. No medical jargon here. It's a quick read that swiftly puts you on the road to recovery from injuries you can generally treat yourself.

From his long experience as the supervising physical therapist at the famed Nicholas Institute of Sports Medicine and Athletic Trauma (NISMAT) in New York City, Benjamin Gel-

fand and coauthor Morton Dean have perfected a "two min-
ute drill" for the aching athlete. It's designed to take you no
longer than two minutes to understand what ails you and
how to deal with it.

Got a problem with a shoulder? Identify the specific ail-
ment in the "Shoulder" section. The leg's gimpy? Turn to the
"Leg" page for treatment strategies. With this handy reference guide, you will be able to identify your distinct problem
from head to toe by matching your pain with the words in
"The Pain" section for every athletic injury.

Instant relief is the goal of every Glory Days jock. "Can I
alleviate the pain?" "Should I elevate my leg?" "How do I
keep the swelling down?" "Should I use ice or heat?" "Do I
apply the ice directly and for how long?" You'll find out
quickly and explicitly in "The First Day Treatment" section,
which describes the program you should follow immediately
during the first twenty-four hours of caring for your injury.

If you have listened to the babble of amateur medical advice from the sidelines when you're hurting, you know there
are conflicting notions about how to respond to many injuries. "Ice it!" "No, put heat on it!" Few weekend warriors are
aware there are potential dangers from misusing ice and
heat. So, we have included strong warnings throughout the
book to prevent you from making bad decisions about treating your particular problem.

For a more detailed understanding of what happened to
your body you'll get "an X-ray view" of each injury by reading "The Inside Story."

On a scale of 1 up to 4, "The Risk Rating" explains the
seriousness of your injury and its long-range outlook if you
ignore the problem.

"When can I return to action?" is the anguished athlete's
innermost concern. The "Return to Action" section has the
answer.

If a period of rehab is necessary, you'll learn exactly what
to do in the "Rehab and Prevention" section.

The book offers expert, descriptive help—including drawings—for rehabilitating the injury so that you regain your health and mobility, and for preventing a recurrence. Prevention is a major element of the book. A program of strengthening and stretching exercises is specifically designed to hasten your return to full power, and to make another hobbling experience less likely.

The exercises relate not only to the specific injury, but to the surrounding muscles as well. It's called *linkage!* It's a concept developed by Dr. James Nicholas, founder of the famous New York sports medicine institute bearing his name. Basically, it's based on the premise that all of the muscles and bones in the human body can be considered as a series of links in a chain. A weakness or injury in one link is likely to adversely affect nearby links. The chain is only as strong as its weakest link. If you tend to favor your painful area, or if a weakness develops there from misuse, the imbalance is likely to produce trouble elsewhere. For example, an ankle sprain often results in a painful hip or back. The reverse can also be true—a weak hip or back can set you up for an ankle injury. Rehabilitating the weak link is imperative to reestablish a proper relationship with the other links. And strengthening the surrounding links is an important way to compensate for any deficits in the chain.

When applicable you'll also find valuable advice about how to avoid aches and pains by making simple choices, such as changing your footwear, deciding on a different playing or running surface, and even changing the size, cut, or fabric of the clothing you wear.

While simplicity is the key throughout the book, all information and recommendations are based on sound sports medicine theories and practices used in top clinics and professional sport training rooms. These theories and practices have been developed by specialists—orthopedists, physical therapists, and athletic trainers—and have been proven to help maximize performance while minimizing injury.

◆ BASIC RULES ◆

WARNINGS, MYTHS, MOTHER'S TALES, AND MISCONCEPTIONS!

1. Ice or heat: The eternal debate! Which one should I use and when?

Ice is always used to minimize swelling and to treat pain associated with it. In most cases, ice is especially important during the first twenty-four to thirty-six hours after an injury. However, while ice can be a Glory Days athlete's best friend, if you exceed the limits suggested for your particular injury, blisters and tissue damage can result.

Heat should be used as directed for pain relief, muscle soreness, and muscle spasms, as well as to promote flexibility. It's important that you follow the specific directions regarding the use of heat for your particular injury. Always use moderate heat. If the heat-induced redness on your skin remains for more than one hour after removing the heat source, it was too hot. An excessive amount of heat applied to an injured area can blister your skin and cause burns requiring emergency medical attention. Also, do not apply heat to treat swelling, as it will just increase the amount of swelling in the injured area.

With advancing age, Glory Days athletes may be more likely to suffer from circulatory problems in their hands and feet. If you have been diagnosed with that problem, seek medical advice about the use of heat and ice in treating your injuries.

2. Is it okay to eat just before exercising?

No! To prevent an upset stomach, always allow two hours between chowing down and gearing up. If you're eating a heavy meal, you might want to wait an extra hour.

3. Mort's mother used to warn her children against swimming soon after eating. "Wait an hour," she would advise. "Otherwise, you'll get cramps and drown!" Was this sound advice?

Yes and no. As above, it's wise to wait at least two hours after eating before swimming for exercise. If you violate the rule you won't drown, but you may get an upset stomach.

4. Your dad's coach probably used to tell him to eat a big steak on the day of the big game. What kind of food is appropriate if you're engaging in a sports competition?

Pasta! You can't go wrong with it. It's high in complex carbohydrates, which are easily digestible and provide a quick source of fuel for your body. If you're a rare person who doesn't like pasta, then bread or rice are good substitutes.

5. Is it important to drink fluids *before* exercising?

Yes. It is essential to fill your tank. Don't overdo it, though. If you're going to sweat a lot, remember that a loss of 2 to 3 percent of your body weight due to dehydration can reduce performance.

6. What kind of fluids are best to take *before* physical activity?

Water is good. But if you plan on going full tilt for more than one hour, a commercially available sports drink, rich in electrolytes, is a better choice. Avoid alcohol.

7. What about drinking liquids *during* physical activity?

It's important to always keep fluid levels in your body constant. During an hour of vigorous activity, as many as three cups of fluid might be necessary to replace what you lost.

8. What kind of fluids are best to drink *during* activity?

Water and, if your activity requires hard work and lasts more than an hour, sports drinks work the best. Avoid fruit juices because they can cause diarrhea during and after intense physical activity.

9. Is it important to drink *after* physical activity?

Absolutely! Replace what you lost. How thirsty you are is not a good indication of how much fluid has to be replaced. Weigh yourself before and after. For each pound you lost, you should drink two cups of fluid, again, either water or a carbohydrate- and electrolyte-rich sports drink. An important reminder: Losing fluids is not the way to lose weight! It's actually quite dangerous to do so, and can cause your body long-term damage.

10. What fluids are best *after* you complete your sporting activity?

Water is okay, but it's best to follow your activity with a sports drink, rich in carbohydrates and electrolytes.

11. What about downing a beer or two during a break in the action?

Never drink alcoholic beverages while you're engaging in athletic activity. Alcohol quickens the dehydration process.

12. What about a coffee break?

Coffee, or other caffeinated beverages, are unlikely to provide any benefits to a Glory Days athlete and can also cause dehydration.

13. **Mort's old high school coach warned against drinking liquids that were too cold. "Room temp," he advised sternly. Does temperature make a difference?**

No! It doesn't matter whether it's hot or cold, as long as you drink up to replenish what your body loses.

14. **Your grandmother frets about women athletes performing during their menstrual periods. Is there any reason for her concern?**

No. Play on!

15. **How important is warming up before physical activity?**

Very. But it doesn't mean just touching your toes ten times. We recommend ten minutes of light jogging, walking, or cycling with a stationary or moving bike followed by gentle stretching. Warming up increases blood flow and the temperature of your muscles, helping them to become more flexible and less prone to injury.

16. **Is it wise to cool down after you finish?**

Yes. It's vital that your heart return to its normal pumping level. So slowly ease off of your physical activity. You can cool down the way you warmed up before you began exercising by doing ten minutes of light jogging, cycling, or walking. The cooling-off period is important because most abnormal rhythms of the heart occur within ten minutes after exercise.

17. **Ben's mother always cautioned against working up a sweat when he wasn't feeling well. Is this wise counsel?**

It depends. If you have flulike symptoms such as muscle aches, fever, chills, diarrhea, or vomiting, sports activity will likely make matters worse. If you have a minor head cold, a stuffy or runny nose, or a simple sore throat, exercise is okay, but monitor yourself and stop if your symptoms get worse. When returning from an illness, start out slowly.

18. Are there any dangers from using an elastic wrap?

If your injury requires the use of an elastic wrap, be alert to the catastrophic potential for cutting off your blood circulation. Loosen it if the area you're treating becomes numb, cold, or begins to throb. Always remove the wrap before you fall asleep!

19. If you're uptight and have had a bad day, is the answer exercise?

Coaches and trainers are not the only ones to vouch for the therapeutic value of athletic activity. Psychiatrists and psychologists now cite an impressive array of research to suggest that mental health, as well as physical well-being, are often enhanced by physical exertion. But remember this: Psychological tension can produce physiological damage. So, before you begin, take a few deep breaths and relax. Tension on the job or at home often leads to muscle tightness, which if not resolved before you exercise, can lead to pulls, spasms, and even breaks.

20. How often should I buy a new pair of athletic shoes? There are so many from which to choose—does it make a difference which ones I purchase?

Too many Glory Days athletes ignore the condition of their athletic shoes. While it doesn't matter whether you have the most expensive pair, it's extremely important that your shoes fit well, provide excellent support, and absorb shock to ease the wear and tear on your legs. It's time to buy a new pair when the treads begin to wear out, even if the wear is limited to just one area of the sole. Also, if either shoe has begun to lose its original shape, it means it's no longer providing the kind of support you need. So, head to the store!

21. Should you immediately resort to painkillers or anti-inflammatories to control your injury?

While this book promotes self-help, the authors fully realize the value of other therapies under specific conditions. Pay special attention to the advice found in the section dealing with your particular injury. There are many medical pros who advocate the use of various medicines to treat sports injuries. Seek good medical counsel if you're considering the use of even over-the-counter remedies. Always read the directions fully and follow them carefully.

22. Is it really important to begin the recommended exercises as soon as possible?

Absolutely. Unused or barely used muscles begin to lose strength within three days. It's important not only to recapture what you had but to improve upon it as well.

Part Two

---◆---

AN INJURY
GUIDE TO
THE
BODY

AN INJURY GUIDE TO THE BODY
(Front)

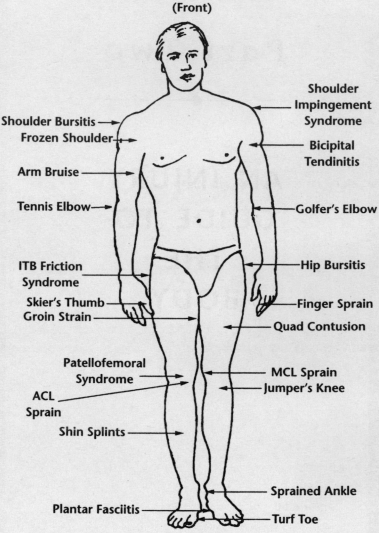

Shoulder Bursitis

Frozen Shoulder

Arm Bruise

Tennis Elbow

ITB Friction
Syndrome

Skier's Thumb

Groin Strain

Patellofemoral
Syndrome

ACL
Sprain

Shin Splints

Plantar Fasciitis

Shoulder
Impingement
Syndrome

Bicipital
Tendinitis

Golfer's Elbow

Hip Bursitis

Finger Sprain

Quad Contusion

MCL Sprain

Jumper's Knee

Sprained Ankle

Turf Toe

AN INJURY GUIDE TO THE BODY
(Back)

Stiff Neck

Trigger
Point

Lower Back
Strain

Carpal Tunnel
Syndrome

Hamstring
Strain

Runner's
Knee

Knee
Arthritis

Calf Strain

Achilles Tendon
Rupture

Achilles
Tendinitis

Part Three

◆

THE
INJURIES

NECK

Stiff Neck

THE PAIN

Something, rather than someone, has given you a pain in the neck. A tightness has developed. You can move your neck in one direction, but not the other. The stiffness—and pain—seem to be radiating down into your shoulder, or up to your head. Or in both directions simultaneously. No big mystery here—you are suffering from a **neck spasm**. An old-fashioned **stiff neck**.

LOCKER ROOM LINGO

"I've got a stiff neck" sounds more like a comment from your childhood than a manifestation of a possible sports injury. Some jocks, fearing exposure as wimps, prefer to complain about having "*a kink*" than a "*stiff neck.*" However, unthreatened Glory Days athletes, secure in their musculature and accomplishments, are more likely than not—in this particular case—to honor tradition. "Stiff neck" is just fine. It's neither déclassé nor delicate, and will not diminish your stature among your peers.

THE INSIDE STORY

Among the many muscles in your neck are the three trapezius: upper, middle, and lower. They travel from the shoulder blade to the vertebrae of the neck, covering your upper and lower back. A stiff neck is usually caused by a spasm—an uncontrolled flexing action—in the upper trapezius.

THE RISK RATING

If not taken care of, this injury can become a nagging problem of recurring stiffness and soreness. The longer the injury is present without treatment, the harder it will be to treat.

THE GAME

A likely scenario: The first deep freeze of the winter has glazed your favorite pond with a slick, thick, shiny, blemish-free covering of ice. The crispness of the day and the mirror

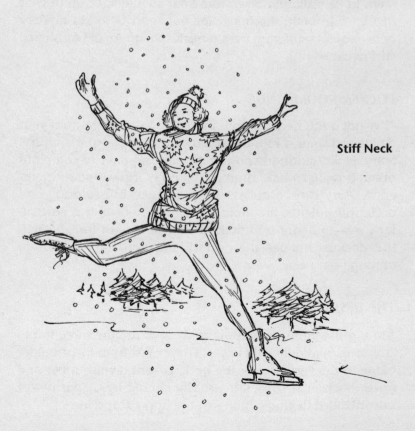

Stiff Neck

reflection of the sun-filled sky is a perfect greeting card of the season. You plan to etch a personal salutation in carefully constructed swirls across the virgin ice. As you lace up your skates, your favorite wool sweater, pungently protected by moth balls and cedar during the off-season, sparks one of those aromatic awakenings. It takes you back through time, long ago, before a childlike pleasure, performed barely beyond the protective reach of a grandparent's hand, turned into an annual adult obsession. The ease with which the sweater conforms loosely to your shape is a pleasant suggestion that time has been charitable, and not all has been lost with the passage of another year. As you sweep out across the ice, gestures more grand by the moment, you attempt to imitate an Olympic-level double lutz. But lutz quickly becomes klutz. There is an aching, ominous instant when something feels wrong—a problem in your neck. And soon it returns. You reach up, massage it with your fingertips, and try the move again. Now you are forced to stop. The pain is severe. So much for the poetry of winter. You have yourself to blame—if only you had warmed up! You ignored the warning that the older you get the more you have to stretch your stiffening muscles and ligaments.

THE FIRST DAY TREATMENT

IMMEDIATE: **Rest It**

It's unwise to continue any athletic activity that hurts your neck. Attempting to play while you are suffering from a stiff neck can only prolong the painful spasms and extend the recovery period.

IMMEDIATE: **Heat It**

As soon as possible, get some heat on the affected area for twenty minutes. During the first twenty-four hours, try to arrange your schedule so that you can repeat the heat application five times during the day, but no more than once an hour. Use a heating pad, a hot pack, or slip into a hot bath.

RETURN TO ACTION

The pain may disappear in one day but could take as long as a week. When the stiffness in your neck has disappeared, you can return to active participation in sports that require upper body movement.

Be on red alert, though. If you have any indication the stiffness is about to recur, stop what you're doing and head for the heat!

REHAB AND PREVENTION

There is no substitute for warming up, not only before you participate in athletic activity, but before you begin a regimen of exercises as well. In a sense, the warm-ups are pre-exercise exercises.

As you participate in the rehab and prevention phase, if your neck still bothers you, apply heat to it for twenty minutes four times a day. If circumstances permit, do not crowd the heat applications into just one part of the day.

After your activity use an ice pack on it for ten minutes, or ice-massage the painful area for five minutes.

The way you're holding your head and neck may need to change. Double-check your alignment. The pillow you sleep on may be too soft and not providing enough support. Or, it could be too hard or too high, creating too stressful an angle. Find the perfect pillow.

REHAB AND PREVENTION REVIEW

◆ Warm it up!
◆ Heat it up!

- ◆ Chill it down!
- ◆ Test your alignment!
- ◆ Buy a new pillow!

▶ **CAUTION:** In all cases, use moderate heat. It's too hot if redness lasts more than one hour after heat application or blisters form.

▶ **CAUTION:** Monitor your icing carefully, as excessive use of ice can cause blisters and skin damage.

▶ **CAUTION:** If you suffer from circulatory problems, seek medical advice about the use of heat or ice.

THE EXERCISES

Neck stretch: 1 ◆ 2 ◆ 3 ◆ 4 ◆ 5 ◆ 6

Trigger Point

THE PAIN

It feels as if something has knotted in your neck. While no swelling is apparent when you look in the mirror, when you probe with your finger, you discover a knot under your skin. It actually feels like a pebble or a marble has somehow lodged itself there. As you apply pressure, the pain can be severe, radiating out from the **trigger point**. The pain might be familiar—possibly you've had a trigger point elsewhere in your body. While they are most common in the neck or upper back, they can occur almost anywhere. If the knot has developed in your neck, it might feel like just another stiff neck. But if you feel that knot, it's a trigger point.

LOCKER ROOM LINGO

In an effort to ease the discomfort, your Glory Days friends see you doing some mambolike movements with your neck, head, and shoulders. "What have you got, a knot?" a pain-experienced jock will ask. A more playful, if not morbid, individual will approach you and jab the knot with a finger. As you cry out in pain, the perpetrator will say in a self-satisfied way, "Hey! Great aim, huh? I zapped the trigger point." **A knot, a trigger point.** That's what you have, and that's what was zapped.

THE INSIDE STORY

Trigger points, from BB to pea size, can appear and disappear suddenly and mysteriously as part of a muscle or ligament anywhere in the body. To the touch they are hard and round, as they are made up of swollen fibers in the muscle or ligament itself. The general belief is that the trigger point erupts from an *inflamed* muscle or ligament, although there is a long, lingering medical controversy about the exact cause.

THE RISK RATING

Be sure to rehab this injury. If not, it can become chronic and disabling.

THE GAME

A likely scenario: Your fantasy has taken you inside the ring, contesting for the World Championship. You're pounding away—jabbing with a left, right, left, left—setting up the opponent for a knockout blow. Suddenly, you're no longer able to slip side-to-side as you jab, and a painful tightening in your neck brings you back to reality, back to the gym, back

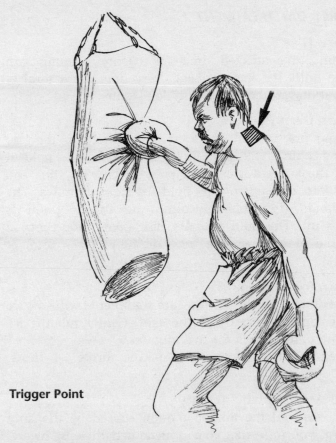

Trigger Point

to the big bag that has barely moved despite an assault from your best punches. Your trainer, a wise old battle-scarred corner man, is now expertly walking his fingers over your neck. When he approaches the trigger point, your knees buckle as if you have just taken a devastating counterpunch from an unseen opponent. You don't remember exactly how the knot developed—was it the swift movement of your fists, the bobbing and weaving of your head and shoulders, or the resistance of the punching bag that has created the problem? It is the nature of trigger points that they seem to just "come on," often without any specific traumatic moments.

THE FIRST DAY TREATMENT

IMMEDIATE: Heat

Heating the affected area for twenty minutes can begin to untie the knot. Repeat every hour for a total of five times during the first twenty-four hours.

IMMEDIATE: Deep Pressure

Putting pressure on the knot is definitely in the "no pain, no gain" category. Take a tennis ball, hold it against the knotted area, and press firmly. Yes, this will hurt. If you can tolerate it, hold for three minutes. The pain should decrease, indicating the trigger point is breaking up. The pain will not disappear altogether, so repeat the pressure process once an hour, for a total of five times.

IMMEDIATE: Ice Massage

Immediately follow the pressure treatments with an ice massage, applied directly to the skin. Gently rub the ice across the painful area for five minutes.

Remember to follow this specific order: 1–HEAT. 2–PRESSURE. 3–ICE.

OPTIONAL: Stop Athletic Activity

The pain and the limited motion caused by the knot may force you to restrict your athletic activities. Be aware! When suffering from knots and pulls, you may try to compensate for the problem by improper body motion, thus causing injury to another muscle or ligament.

RETURN TO ACTION

It's smart to wait for the acute pain to diminish before putting the knotted area to the test. When you have a minimal amount of pain you can ease back into your regular athletic activities. If there were a pain meter for the neck, minimal would equal a 3 on a scale of 1 to 10 of increasing severity.

Take care in testing your limits. Knots frequently return to bedevil even the best-conditioned Glory Days jocks.

REHAB AND PREVENTION

For the neck, especially, good habits can often deter bad problems. Try to improve your posture. Be conscious of it at all times, not only when you're involved in athletic activity. Just a slight alteration in your body movement during physical activity can eliminate a likely cause of your problem. A pro can often spot what's wrong and help you adjust as you throw a punch, swing a bat or racquet, or bounce down the roadway during your daily jog.

Psychological tension often produces physiological damage. Tension on the job or at home often leads to muscle tightness, which can lead to pulls, spasms, and breaks if not resolved before you exercise. Relax. Take a few deep breaths.

Once you have suffered this injury, be especially certain to warm up before engaging in your favorite athletic activity. Doing the neck stretches listed below will help.

If you feel that the trigger points are returning, ice the area. Cool it with an ice pack for ten minutes.

REHAB AND PREVENTION REVIEW

- ♦ Stretch!
- ♦ Ice!
- ♦ Warm up!
- ♦ Master your mechanics!
- ♦ Perfect your posture!
- ♦ Relieve tension!

► CAUTION: Use moderate heat. It's too hot if redness lasts more than one hour after heat application or if blisters form.

► CAUTION: Excessive use of ice can cause blisters or skin damage.

▶ CAUTION: If you suffer from circulatory problems, seek medical advice about the use of heat or ice.

THE EXERCISES

Neck stretch: 1 ◆ 2 ◆ 3 ◆ 4 ◆ 5 ◆ 6

Shoulder Impingement

THE PAIN

As you lift your arm you feel a dull ache on the side of, or just below, your shoulder. Sometimes it feels as if there's a tack in your shoulder that presses into the muscle and bone when you try to lift your arm. It's not just a swift athletic movement that causes the pain. The discomfort is felt when you put on a jacket, reach around to scratch your back, or even while trying to pick out a best-seller from the top shelf of a bookstore. You're experiencing the kind of discomfort associated with **shoulder impingement syndrome.** A problem with your **rotator cuff.**

LOCKER ROOM LINGO

In the locker room, the problem is simply called the **tator** or the **cuff.**

THE INSIDE STORY

When you lift your arm there is a tug-of-war of sorts between two muscle groups, the deltoids and the rotator cuff. The deltoids consist of three parts that are responsible for lifting your arm in front of your body, lifting your arm out to the side, and moving your arm horizontally backwards. The rotator cuff muscles rotate your arm inward and outward, and also help the deltoids do their job. If there's a weakness in the rotator cuff group, a tendon attached to one of those muscles (the supraspinatus) is being pinched between the arm bone (the humerus) and the shoulder bone (the acromion process).

Natural blood flow in your body contributes to healing. Because there is little blood in this area, once it's damaged, it is unlikely to heal quickly.

THE RISK RATING

Rotator cuff injuries strike fear into pro quarterbacks and pitchers for good reason. If not rehabilitated, the tator injury can progress to a tear. A small hole might even develop. This more severe injury is unlikely to heal on its own, and surgery might be needed. So it's important for you to not overlook the early symptoms, because the odds are they will not go away on their own and will worsen with use.

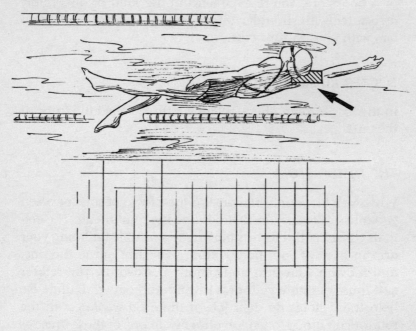

Shoulder Impingement

THE GAME

A likely scenario: You dive into the cool water for the first swim of the summer. A confident swimmer, you begin the overhead motions that propel you through the water. After a few minutes you begin to feel an ache in the shoulder or on the side of your arm. The pain is evident with each stroke you take. Back on the beach, and eager to pump up your muscles after a lazy winter, you begin a fast-moving game of kadima, which entails paddling a ball back and forth with a friend. Every time you reach for a high ball, that pain you felt while swimming returns and intensifies. You lie on a blanket hoping the hot sun will bake the pain away, but each time you lift your arm to rub on sunscreen, you are disappointed.

THE FIRST DAY TREATMENT

IMMEDIATE: **Stop Any Activity That Produces Pain**
To prevent further damage and possible lengthening of the rehab period, try not to perform any task requiring that you lift your arm above the shoulder.

IMMEDIATE: **Stop All Heavy Lifting**
Whether or not you experience pain, you should refrain from all strenuous lifting.

RETURN TO ACTION

Wait until the ache subsides. This could take several weeks.

REHAB AND PREVENTION

If you attack the problem early on, you might succeed in getting the "tator" back in shape quickly and easily.

During the rehab process try not to lift your arm above your shoulder. Let someone else do the heavy lifting. If your sport is swimming, you might try adjusting the overhead arm movements that propel you through the water. If tennis or racquetball is your sport, adjusting your serve and overhead swing might help eliminate the pain. You can adapt on your own or ask a pro for a lesson.

However, the cause of your pain might be muscular weakness. As a result, you might move your shoulder incorrectly. Often this can be resolved by exercise to strengthen the rotator cuff muscles.

Remember, put an ice pack on the "tator," or massage it with ice for fifteen minutes after each rehab session. Follow that advice after you have returned to your sport as well.

REHAB AND PREVENTION REVIEW

◆ Restrict arm and shoulder movements!
◆ Avoid pain!
◆ Evaluate the cause!
◆ Strengthen!
◆ Stretch!
◆ Ice!

▶ CAUTION: Remember that excessive use of ice can cause blisters and skin damage.

THE EXERCISES

Shoulder strengthen: 1 ◆ 2 ◆ 5 ◆ 6 ◆ 7

Elbow strengthen: 1

Shoulder stretch: 1 ◆ 2

Frozen Shoulder

THE PAIN

You try to move your arm but your shoulder won't respond the way you want it to. It appears to be locked in place. It's as if some of its elasticity is gone. How did this happen? You probably recall that the top and side of your shoulder hurt. You felt pain not only when you reached high or wide during an athletic endeavor but when you reached into your back pocket, slipped into your jacket, brushed your hair, or smoothed suspenders or a bra strap behind your back. Not willing to experience that kind of pain again, you began to limit your shoulder movements. But now, even when you try to use your full range of motion, you can't do so. Your shoulder won't respond beyond a certain point. The problem could have been caused originally by a response to pain from a rotator cuff injury, shoulder bursitis (refer to sections about these injuries), or by a broken arm that required you to use a sling. This is a clearly defined case of **adhesive capsulitis**.

LOCKER ROOM LINGO

Frozen shoulder. But remember, it has nothing to do with the weather or temperature.

THE INSIDE STORY

Your troubled shoulder joint (the glenohumeral) is surrounded by a glove of synovial membranes that provide nutrition and stability. Like an accordion, they have folds that give you the ability to move and to reach out. If you don't use it, you lose it! The longer you immobilize your shoulder, the number of folds losing their elasticity increases.

THE RISK RATING

Failure to follow rehab advice could result in a long-term problem, possibly costing you severe shoulder difficulties up to a year or longer. Rehab it! It's a must!

THE GAME

A likely scenario: The recuperation period is over. Or so you think. After being out of action because of a shoulder problem, you are ready to tone up by pumping iron. Yes, you have noticed problems in performing some of your ADLs (the activities of daily living), but you're certain the full use of your shoulder will return if you push through and give that

Frozen Shoulder

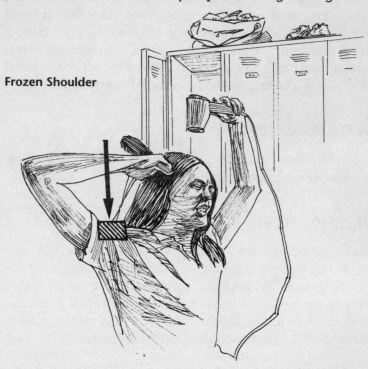

side of your body more muscle power. The experience is frustrating. The weight compounds your difficulty and reconfirms how much shoulder motion you have lost.

THE FIRST DAY TREATMENT

IMMEDIATE: **Stop, But Don't Immobilize**

Avoid all painful movements of that shoulder. However, it's extremely important to keep it as mobile as possible to prevent further limitation of motion. This may seem contradictory. It's not. The key is to avoid using the muscles on top of your shoulder (the deltoids) on the troubled side. So, extend your range of motion—step by step, just beyond the point of pain—by moving your shoulder passively, that is, by giving it some help with your other arm or a pulley. Hold that position for five seconds. Do a set of fifty pulls, three times during the first twenty-four hours. Wait at least an hour between sets.

IMMEDIATE: Ice

Ice the painful area for twenty minutes. Repeat the icing if the pain returns.

IMMEDIATE: **Get the Pendulum Swinging**

The exercises designed to maintain or increase your shoulder's ROM—range of motion—are the pendulums, which, like all required exercises, are described in the exercise section of the book. While there is some evidence ROM will eventually improve on its own in about nine months, you can accelerate your recovery by *immediately* devoting yourself to the pendulums.

RETURN TO ACTION

Frozen shoulder can put a freeze on some of your athletic activities for at least two weeks. A severe case will keep you on the shelf for up to six months. Ben's test for a safe return is the pain-free moving of your arms over your head, behind your head, and moving your arms behind your back. Obviously you can—at any time—perform athletic activities that don't cause you any shoulder pain.

REHAB AND PREVENTION

Before each R&P session, put heat on the bad shoulder for twenty minutes.

Stretching is not an option in dealing with frozen shoulder. It's a must! Perform these exercises diligently. Building up the strength of the shoulder and elbow is an important preventive measure.

An important note: While performing this rehab and prevention regimen, you will likely experience some pain for a while. In this case, it's beneficial pain—it means you're undoing your problem. However, any pain outside this narrowly defined plan is to be avoided.

Only after you have completed an R&P session, ice the shoulder for ten minutes. It should help alleviate any pain.

REHAB AND PREVENTION REVIEW

◆ Put the heat on!
◆ Stretch it out!
◆ Strengthen it up!
◆ No pain, no gain!
◆ Cool it!

▶ CAUTION: Use moderate heat. It's too hot if redness lasts more than one hour after heat application, or if blisters form.

▶ CAUTION: Excessive use of ice can cause blisters or skin damage.

THE EXERCISES

Shoulder stretch: 1 ◆ 2 ◆ 6 ◆ 7 ◆ 8

Shoulder strengthen: 1 ◆ 2 ◆ 5 ◆ 6 ◆ 7

Elbow strengthen: 1

Shoulder Bursitis

THE PAIN

The top part of your arm hurts. The pain is centered where the arm joins the shoulder. The sensitive area may be a bit red, swollen, and feel warm to the touch. It's the kind of pain that you imagine would force a major league baseball pitcher to go on the disabled list. If you imitate the movements of a pitcher throwing a ball, it's likely the pain will increase just as your arm comes up over your head. And the pain will no doubt revisit you when you bring your arm back down by your side. Heavy lifting, such as playfully trying to hoist a young child for a pretend plane ride, is guaranteed to result in an emergency landing. As you have probably noticed, the intermittent shoulder pain can interrupt your plans for a good night's sleep. Finding a comfortable, pain-free position as you prepare for dreamland is not easy. And once you are asleep, any tossing and turning of your upper body will serve as an unwelcome wake-up call. You are suffering from **shoulder bursitis.**

Note: Some of these symptoms are reminiscent of the infamous rotator cuff problem that is described in the section devoted to that injury.

LOCKER ROOM LINGO

The frame of reference depends on your sport. Pitch, and it's a **pitcher's shoulder.** Swim, and it's **swimmer's shoulder.** In many locker rooms, simplicity suffices. It's just a **shoulder burr.**

THE INSIDE STORY

The burr refers to the bursa. It's a fluid-filled sac made of tissue that helps to minimize friction between the top of the arm bone (the humerus) and the lower end of the shoulder bone (the acromion process). The fluid within the bursa is called synovium. When there's muscle weakness in the shoulder, the sac becomes pinched between the arm bone and the shoulder bone. That irritation of the bursa causes the body to produce more synovial fluid, enlarging the size of the bursa and adding to your misery.

THE RISK RATING

Failure to take corrective measures could lead to another problem—frozen shoulder—with potentially longer lasting complications.

THE GAME

A likely scenario: You're on the mound. Each time when you deliver the ball toward home plate you feel a tinge in your shoulder. The feeling has been there before, but is increasing in frequency and intensity. When you step away from the plate to prepare your next pitch, the pain travels with you. Later, it hurts when you towel down, when you try to reach around to soap up your back in the shower, and even when you take a deep breath and try to relax your body. You wonder when you'll be able to get back into the swing of things.

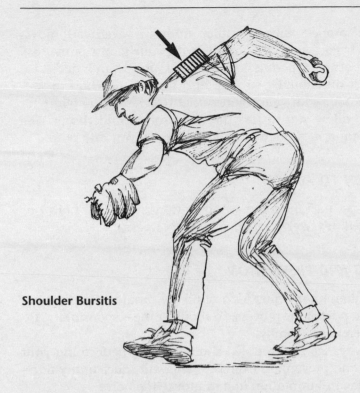

Shoulder Bursitis

THE FIRST DAY TREATMENT

IMMEDIATE: Brr the Burr

Massage the shoulder with ice as soon as you can after feeling the pain. A five-minute massage should restrict the inflammation and diminish the pain. Place the ice directly on the shoulder and rub it across the painful area. One ice massage is not enough. Ben's rule: five ice massages in the first twenty-four hours.

IMMEDIATE: Avoid Pain-causing Movements

If you return to the pool or the playing fields before the pain is completely gone, be smart! Don't risk further injury. If you can't stay out of the pool, use the dog pad-

dle to propel yourself rather than an overhead movement. If you want to continue with your tennis game, ask
your partner's permission to serve underhand and take
no over-the-shoulder strokes. In a friendly baseball or softball game, your teammates might feel sorry enough for
you to allow you to toss the ball around underhand. The
underhand movement should not cause you any pain.

RETURN TO ACTION

Don't get back into the swing of things until all pain has
subsided. It's likely to take at least six weeks.

REHAB AND PREVENTION

Strengthening the muscles around the shoulder is a very important part of the process. So shoulder the responsibility. Do
the exercises faithfully.

Always ice the troubled shoulder after performing your
rehab and prevention exercises. This will squelch any flare-
up of the inflammation and minimize the pain.

Do not perform any rehab and prevention activities that
cause pain.

If you have been swimming with hand paddles to
strengthen your arms and shoulders . . . **stop.** It aggravates
the condition.

REHAB AND PREVENTION REVIEW

◆ Strengthen!
◆ Ice!
◆ Check your technique!
◆ Limit activity!

▶ CAUTION: Excessive use of ice can cause blisters and skin
damage.

THE EXERCISES

Shoulder stretch: 1 ◆ 2 ◆ 6

Shoulder strengthen: 2 ◆ 4 ◆ 5 ◆ 6

Elbow strengthen: 1 ◆ 2

BACK

Lower Back Strain

THE PAIN

"Oh, my aching back!" has become the moaning mantra that permeates your day. Just a slight shift in your posture elevates the intensity of the pain on one or both sides of the lower back just above your waistline. The discomfort may be apparent even as you gently run your hand over the area, or try to massage it with your fingertips. You grope for words to describe your back problem. "A dull pain that suddenly becomes sharp as if I were stabbed with a knife. . . ." "A throbbing sensation. . . ." "It feels as if my whole back is about to 'go out'. . . ." "It's as if one side of my back has become unhinged and locked in place. . . ." "It began as a little localized ache but has widened and worsened. . . ." "My back has gone out!" Just about any athletic activity—bending over to grab a ground ball, sidestepping the mast to change directions while windsurfing, doing a racing turn in the pool—generates pain no matter how delicately you try to maneuver. If your sport requires lacing up a shoe, you'll probably get the message before you even begin to participate. Pay attention to the message! Even if you believe you can play through the pain, it's too risky. You are suffering from **mechanical low back** pain, a sprain or strain of your muscles or ligaments.

▶ WARNING: If you feel a severe pain that radiates from your back down below your belt to your butt or legs, or if you can't sit for more than a few minutes without the pain increasing, it's likely your problem is more serious than mechanical low back pain. The possibilities include a herniated or slipped disc, and sciatica, which require medical attention.

LOCKER ROOM LINGO

You can call it "B.S."! Not B.S. as a descriptive way of discrediting your complaint, but B.S. for **Back Syndrome!** If you don't want to b.s. your Glory Days colleagues, simply tell them you're suffering from "lower back pain" or have "thrown" your back out. Unless they live in a world of macho denial (as in, "I just don't *understand* pain"), they will react knowingly and sympathetically.

THE INSIDE STORY

The back is an essential component of almost every movement your body makes. It acts as the stability point for movement of your arms, legs, and head. Among the muscles in your back are the erector spinae. Long and thin, they act as antigravity muscles that keep your body from collapsing. They run from head to tail, connecting with the vertebrae located at the base of your skull and those just above your butt. These back muscles have to be treated with care; otherwise, you'll develop mechanical low back pain.

THE RISK RATING

If you continue to play you will continue to pay! Unattended this problem can become chronic.

THE GAME

A likely scenario: You're in the gym toning your muscles. With the confidence of someone whose mirror has already reflected what you perceive as the reemerging of your sculpted Glory Days shape, you bend your knees, straighten your back, wrap your fingers around a cold steel barbell, take

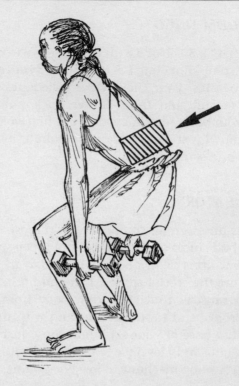

Mechanical Lower Back Strain

a deep breath, and lift. The ego surge is momentary. A swift, sharp pain cuts across your lower back—as if you have just been attacked with a samurai sword. The excruciating peak of the pain goes away as quickly as it comes, but not before you reflexively release the barbell, which clangs to the floor, nearly crushing your toes and ruining your new, aerodynamically designed sneakers that cost you the price of a dinner at a five-star French countryside inn. As you straighten up slowly, you're acutely aware that this will be a short night at the gym. There is a residual ache in your back, and you sense that at any moment you may again be visited by the samurai.

THE FIRST DAY TREATMENT

IMMEDIATE: **Stop Painful Activity**

If your back begins to hurt—no matter what the intensity—**stop the painful activity.** If the pain has forced you to your knees or flat onto the floor, try to relax and become as comfortable as possible. Back off from any activity that causes pain in your back. Example: Wear loafers if tying your shoes is painful.

The floor is a perfect place to wait out the pain and relieve the pressure. Lie flat, except for your knees. Put a pillow or two under your knees to elevate them, and stay in that position until the pain decreases or you feel comfortable enough to move. If the pain is very severe, you'll probably need help to get you where you want to go.

Spend the night on a firm surface. Put a board under your mattress or use the floor. Try to keep the knees elevated.

IMMEDIATE: **Heat the Painful Area**

Heat is essential. Twenty minutes of moderate heat should begin to ease the pain. Repeat a total of five times during the day. Ben does not usually recommend heat-generating gels, liniments, or ointments as a first line of defense, because they don't address the problem directly. A heating pad does the trick. But if you choose to soak in a hot bath, be extremely careful as you maneuver your back to get in and out of the tub.

Ben's twenty-four-hour "gut check" comes into play with this injury. If after twenty-four hours the pain continues to immobilize you, you'll probably WANT your doctor to be called, even though your condition is not likely to deteriorate while toughing it out by yourself.

RETURN TO ACTION

Only when your back pain has disappeared **completely** should you resume your normal activities.

REHAB AND PREVENTION

This is a simple, yet profound precaution: Avoid sporting activities that cause pain in your back. If not, you run the risk of generating a chronic problem. As soon as you feel back pain, prepare to work on it so that it will not become a recurring problem.

Whether lifting weights, or lifting children, correct body mechanics are essential. One basic rule: When reaching down to lift anything, **always** bend your knees. Stand close to the object being lifted so you don't have to reach *out* for it.

When shoveling snow (or anything else) bend your knees, **keep your back straight,** and do not twist your back while lifting the shovel. When tying your sneakers or shoes, lift your foot up as high as possible toward your hands rather than bending over.

When sitting, place a rolled towel or pillow across the small of your back and against the back of the chair. The roll should be as wide as your back, and at least four inches thick. It will help you maintain proper posture and should help relieve and prevent pain. This is especially important on long trips: Try it while driving or during an airplane trip! If you prefer, replace the towels with a "lumbar roll," which is commercially available.

Trim any excess weight you may be carrying in your stomach. A big belly alters the alignment of the back and puts added stress on it.

Heat the problem area for fifteen minutes each day before beginning the rehab program.

REHAB AND PREVENTION REVIEW

- ◆ Use correct body mechanics when bending or lifting!
- ◆ Support your lower back!
- ◆ Heat the painful area!
- ◆ Strengthen!

- ♦ Stretch!
- ♦ Trim your front porch!

▶ CAUTION: If your skin remains reddened for more than an hour after the application of heat, you're damaging your skin. Better cool it next time!

THE EXERCISES

Hip strengthen: 1 ♦ 3 ♦ 5

Abdomen strengthen: 1 ♦ 2 ♦ 3 ♦ 4

Back strengthen: 1 ♦ 2 ♦ 3 ♦ 4

Hip and thigh stretch: 1 ♦ 3 ♦ 4

Back stretch: 1 ♦ 2 ♦ 3

Bicipital Tendinitis

THE PAIN

The pain, located just above the muscle of your arm and possibly extending into your shoulder, has come on gradually. First, it was a minor annoyance. Then it became a continuous pain. It aches more when you lift your arm above the shoulder. While pulling a shirt or sweater over your head is a painful experience, it also hurts when you rub your fingers across the area. You have a biceps problem. Doctors call it **bicipital tendinitis**.

LOCKER ROOM LINGO

Any devotee of the macho arts knows where and what the biceps are. Merely saying that you have **biceps tendinitis** is usually enough of a description. But, "Oh, my aching arm muscle" will also make the point.

THE INSIDE STORY

Two distinct muscles make up the biceps muscle group. One is called the long head of the biceps. The other is called the short head of the biceps. Like all other muscles, these two have tendons on either end that attach to bones. Your problem is one of the tendons of the long head. That tendon attaches to the biceps muscle by traveling from the shoulder through the bicipital groove in the arm bone (the humerus). The tendon has been overstressed and overused, like a rope that's been used so often it's begun to lose its strength. In this case, the rope or tendon became inflamed, and possibly has suffered from microtears.

THE RISK FACTOR

Ignore the stretching exercises at your peril! You might suffer even more loss of motion, resulting in what's known as frozen shoulder.

THE GAME

A likely scenario: Short-sleeve and bathing-suit weather is fast approaching. A quick look in the mirror finds the naked body staring back at you less impressive than what you

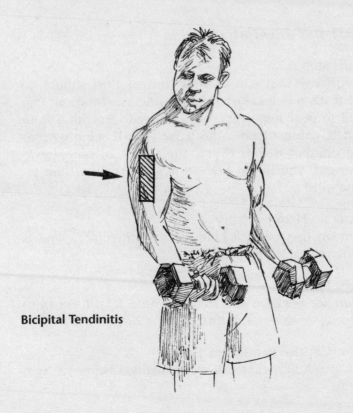

Bicipital Tendinitis

thought would meet the eye. You've got some toning up to do. The barbells are brought out of the closet, and you're back trying to fulfill the oft-broken promise of regular exercise. After a few days, you graduate to twenty-pounders in each hand, lifting them from waist to shoulder, rhythmically, to the beat of your favorite rock album. After about a week of daily pump-'em-up sessions, your concentration is interrupted by a twinge in your upper arm. The more you try to muscle your way through the pain, the worse it feels. Returning to ten-pound weights does not eliminate the discomfort. It's not necessarily the weight that causes the pain—you're just overdoing it! You're causing inflammation by overusing that tendon!

THE FIRST DAY TREATMENT

IMMEDIATE: **Stop**

Any activity that causes your arm to hurt should be avoided if it's painful. Reaching up and reaching out can only add to your rehab time. If you need something from a top shelf, ask a friend to do it for you. If the answer is no, find another friend. If you can't find anyone else to help you out, you might have a bigger problem than biceps tendinitis!

IMMEDIATE: **No Heavy Lifting**

We mean the physical kind. The psychological kind is okay, unless that pains you, too.

IMMEDIATE: **Ice**

Put an ice pack on the troubled area for fifteen minutes. Repeat three times during the first day.

IMMEDIATE: **Get the Pendulum Going**

Begin pendulum exercises recommended below as soon as possible.

RETURN TO ACTION

With appropriate rest and rehabilitation you should be back in the biceps-building business in about four weeks. By then you should be pain free. Do not return until the pain is completely gone!

REHAB AND PREVENTION

Heat the affected area for ten minutes before you begin your R&P program.

To improve your range of motion (ROM), the pendulum exercises begun during the first twenty-four hours of treatment should be continued. It's important to strengthen all the muscles of your arm. As you work on your shoulder, elbow, and forearm, one of the benefits will be that toned-up look you desired in the first place.

As is the case with most injuries, stretching is an extremely important part of the R&P process.

Each session is incomplete without a five-minute ice massage. It's vital during rehab and even later when you have returned to your athletic endeavors. This will reduce inflammation and pain. Remember, when you massage with ice, the ice cube must be rubbed **across** the pain.

This injury is almost always due to overstress. So take it slowly when you return to any form of heavy lifting. If you're lifting weights, proceed slowly toward your goal by gradually increasing the weight. If carrying heavy items is part of your job, and you can make several trips instead of one, do so!

REHAB AND PREVENTION REVIEW

- ◆ Heat!
- ◆ Stretch!
- ◆ Strengthen!
- ◆ Take it slow!

- ◆ ROM!
- ◆ Ice massage!

THE EXERCISES

Shoulder stretch: 1 ◆ 2 ◆ 3 ◆ 8 (pendulum)

Shoulder strengthen: 1 ◆ 2 ◆ 4 ◆ 5 ◆ 6 ◆ 8

Elbow strengthen: 1

Forearm strengthen: 2

Arm Bruise

THE PAIN

The front of your arm hurts about halfway up, between your elbow and shoulder. The pain is very localized, intensifies when you touch it, and you may have difficulty trying to straighten your arm. After a day or two, the area may have swelled and turned black and blue. You have a **contusion.**

LOCKER ROOM LINGO

There should be no contusion confusion. It's an all-purpose, fancy name for a **bruise.** So simply explain to the bruisers you hang out with that's what you have.

THE INSIDE STORY

As soon as you suffer a bad bump or blow, your body responds in a complex and sometimes extraordinary way. Usually swelling and bleeding occur between the injured muscles (the biceps brachii and brachialis brachii) of your arm, and between the bone (the humerus) and the muscles. But sometimes there is a complication. The body can also respond by developing calcium and bone in the damaged muscle fibers. It's that buildup of blood, swelling, calcium, or bone that causes the pain. It's as if a wedge has been placed in the hinge of a swinging door, limiting its motion.

THE RISK RATING

While a bruise might not seem like a big deal, there is a surprisingly strong risk of greater injury if you fail to act quickly or rush your return without following rehab and prevention guidelines.

THE GAME

A likely scenario: The plan was for a fun-filled game of touch football open to all the gals and guys at the office. Despite agreement on rules that would limit the potential for injury, you could predict which co-worker, awash in beer and testosterone (always a dangerous combination for *any* athletic competition), would be unable to distinguish between playfulness and recklessness. As you gracefully sprint to catch a pass, the office ogre, laughingly mocking your physical stature, matches you step for step. Going up for the ball, an elbow crashes into your arm. The pain is instant. Soon you have trouble extending your arm. Reluctant to appear submissive, you refuse to head for the sidelines. You play on. Not a wise idea!

THE FIRST DAY TREATMENT

IMMEDIATE: **Ice It**

Icing this injury is essential. It will quickly reduce pain, swelling, and inflammation. Do it for twenty minutes every four hours during the first day.

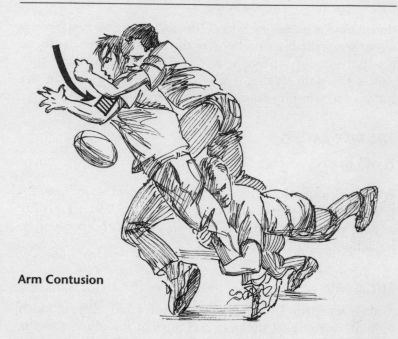

Arm Contusion

▶ CAUTION: Remember that excessive use of ice can cause blisters and skin damage.

IMMEDIATE: **Stop Any Painful Activity**

While the pain might not be substantial, don't try to play through it. If you're eager to compete, play a position that doesn't require the use of your injured arm.

IMMEDIATE: **Compress It**

An elastic wrap can also be used to help reduce the swelling and inflammation.

▶ CAUTION: Remove the wrap before you go to sleep! Be certain it does not cut off circulation.

RETURN TO ACTION

It depends on the severity of the bruise. Plan on a few days to a few weeks. If you have pain and stiffness don't return to your sport until the stiffness is gone.

REHAB AND PREVENTION

▶ CAUTION: Being too aggressive and eager to restore your arm's full range of motion (ROM) can cause more damage and further limit motion. As part of the therapy you must bend and straighten your arm as often as you can, but do it slowly and gently. Do not push it past the point of feeling pain.

Even though your injury was caused by someone else, it's important to strengthen your arm to prevent reinjury. The more muscle mass, the more likely you are to withstand a potentially punishing blow and retain your ability to move your arm without pain. Perform the rehab and prevention exercises! It will save you trouble later on.

Once you return to your normal athletic activities, you might want to wear a pad over the injured area. Other than the obvious protection it provides, it might also give you added confidence that you can play without risk of reinjury.

REHAB AND PREVENTION REVIEW

◆ Slow-mo ROM!
◆ Strengthen!
◆ Pad your part!

THE EXERCISES

Elbow strengthen: 1 ◆ 2

Shoulder strengthen: 1

Forearm strengthen: 1 ◆ 2

Tennis Elbow

THE PAIN

Your elbow aches no matter what you do. The most basic activities, such as squeezing a tube of toothpaste, turning a doorknob, and lifting a shirt from a chest of drawers, are all painful experiences. Your elbow even hurts when touched. When you attempt to grip a tennis racquet to artfully return a hard-hit ground stroke with a backhand, the pain is like an electric shock that moves through the elbow and down the thumb side of your forearm. Welcome to a classic case of *lateral* epicondylitis.

Note: If the pain is on the pinkie finger side of your forearm, refer to the section on Golfer's Elbow (*medial* **epicondylitis**).

LOCKER ROOM LINGO

No matter what caused that pain in the elbow, the most popular and preferred name of the malady is **tennis elbow**. It's a condition that can develop from a variety of athletic and non-sports-related activities, including carrying heavy bags and pulling out roots while gardening. But calling the symptoms "bellboy's elbow" or "gardener's elbow" does not match the athletic aura of **"tennis elbow."**

THE INSIDE STORY

The pain is caused by a tear or inflammation where a tendon (the common extensor tendon) connects a group of muscles to the elbow. The muscles are like rubber bands, and the pain occurs when they have been stretched beyond their capacity and have begun to pull the tendon away from the elbow. These muscles connect at the other end to a variety of tendons that attach to your wrist and fingers. While the pain is always felt in the elbow, it can be caused by improper use of the elbow, fingers, or wrist.

THE RISK RATING

The pain just won't go away on its own. You must rehabilitate it!

THE GAME

A likely scenario: A long-planned weekend of tennis is in full swing as you take on some old friends in a challenging series of matches distinguished more by exuberance than skill. Late in the day you begin to feel a slight soreness on the elbow of your racquet arm. At rest, the arm feels okay, but as you sweep across the court and reach out to accept a volley, the sting is powerful and the more you play, the more the ache tends to linger longer and longer.

THE FIRST DAY TREATMENT

IMMEDIATE: **Rest**

It's imperative not to elbow your way back into action. Give it a rest. Do not try to play through the pain—you risk a much more damaging injury and an extensive rehab period.

IMMEDIATE: **Ice**

Ice should be used to massage your painful elbow for five minutes. Gently rub a cube across the affected area. Do it as soon as possible after feeling the injury, four times during that first day.

Tennis Elbow

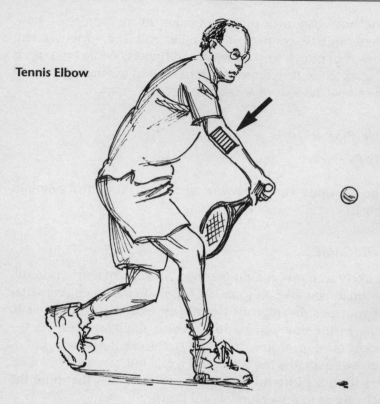

OPTIONAL: **Splint It**

There are many different kinds of splints for sports injuries. The one you should consider has two names: the "cock up" and the "wrist extension." Even though the packaging these splints come in might not refer to tennis elbow, they will relieve some of the tension on the inflamed tendon. Wear it as often as possible, even at night. Be certain it's loose enough so that your circulation is not cut off.

RETURN TO ACTION

Only when you are symptom free! Under normal circumstances it could take four to six weeks if rehabbed properly.

REHAB AND PREVENTION

Get into the rehab habit. There's a lot of work to be done to help solve your elbow problem. But the results will be worth it.

Each time before putting that elbow back to use in a sporting activity, warm it up. Apply heat using a hot-water bottle, a heating pad, or a towel repeatedly soaked in hot water and then placed over your elbow. Do it for ten minutes.

After you've completed every workout, go to the other extreme. Ice the elbow by massaging it directly with an ice cube for five minutes. The ice massage is essential not only after sporting activities but whenever you have put significant pressure on your elbow. Example: If you're on the road again and are carrying your own luggage, order a bucket of ice from room service. Not for a pain-killing martini but to chill your elbow. Another example: If you have a green thumb as well as an aching elbow, follow each trip to the flower bed with a trip to the icebox. If your elbow feels susceptible to further injury, or if it aches at all over the next three months, continue to follow the ice massage routine.

Another type of massage is also very beneficial—the deep friction massage. Rub the painful area firmly with your index and middle fingers for four minutes. Repeat five times a day until the pain disappears.

We also suggest a tension check. Visit a pro shop to determine whether the tension on your racquet strings might be sending unnecessary shock waves up into your elbow.

Getting the right grip on your racquet is not only essential to good performance but can also affect the health of your elbow. So, while you're visiting a pro, ask whether the size of your grip should be modified.

If you play racquet sports, the use of a commercially available countertension strap around your forearm might help absorb some of the shock from hitting the ball.

Until the pain disappears, continue to wear the splint

mentioned in the First Day Treatment section. However, do not wear it on the court when you return to your favorite racquet sport. Note: Do not confuse the "splint" with the "strap."

You've got some work to do on a regular basis even before the pain goes away. You must stretch and strengthen not only your elbow but your wrist and shoulder as well. If any stretching or strengthening exercise causes additional pain, avoid doing that particular exercise, at least temporarily. Return to it only when it can be done pain free.

REHAB AND PREVENTION REVIEW

◆ Heat!
◆ Ice!
◆ Massage!
◆ Stretch!
◆ Strengthen!
◆ Get a good grip on!
◆ Tension check!
◆ Strap it!
◆ Splint it!

▶ CAUTION: Always use moderate heat. It's too hot if redness lasts more than one hour after heat application or blisters form.

▶ CAUTION: Excessive use of ice can cause blisters or skin damage.

THE EXERCISES

Wrist strengthen: 1 ◆ 2

Shoulder strengthen: 5 ◆ 6

Forearm strengthen: 1 ◆ 2

Wrist stretch: 1

Golfer's Elbow

THE PAIN

It began as a slight discomfort on the inside of your elbow, in that part closest to your body. You notice it now each time you bend or straighten your arm, and it is painful when you press on it. If ignored, it gradually becomes more painful whether you're taking a swing, tossing a ball, or tossing down a few drinks to salute that day's athletic achievements. Even bending your elbow to perform a military-style salute causes you to wince. It's easy to produce the pain when you move your elbow, but it's not easy to pronounce the medical name for what ails you. *Medial* **epicondylitis!** (Me-dee-al ehp-ee-con-dih-light-ihs.)

Note: This is different from tennis elbow *(lateral* **epicondylitis)**, which afflicts a different location on your elbow. If your pain is on the *thumb* side of your forearm, refer to the section on tennis elbow.

LOCKER ROOM LINGO

Golfer's elbow or **pitcher's elbow.** If you're neither a golfer nor a pitcher, take your pick!

THE INSIDE STORY

The pain is caused by a tear or inflammation where a tendon (the common flexor tendon) connects the flexor muscles to your elbow. At the other end the flexors connect to a variety of tendons that attach to your wrist and fingers. These muscles help your wrist and palm bend downward and also help bend your fingers. Poor technique in the use of your wrist or elbow can cause tendinitis by putting excessive stress on the tendons that attach to the pinkie finger side of your elbow.

THE RISK RATING

 ①❷③④

If you don't address the problem, you risk more intense pain and a longer convalescence.

THE GAME

A likely scenario: The eighteenth hole is a pleasant sight to you. Not because of any previous luck you've had in approaching the green but because of an annoying pain in your elbow as you swing your clubs. You feel it mostly as you swing downward, powerfully addressing the ball on the tee. Not only do you feel it when you tee off, but also when you

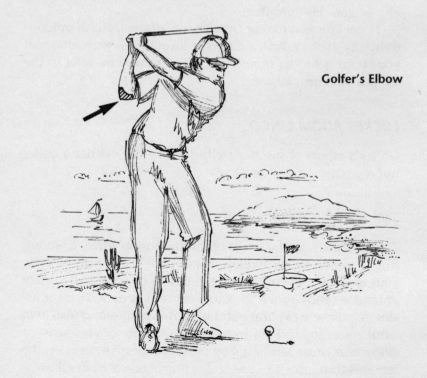

Golfer's Elbow

embarrassingly hit a divot. As the pain worsens during your game, so does your score. In a game that requires concentration, it's not the game on which you begin to concentrate. It's your elbow. Dejectedly, you heft your golf bag and slide your arm under the strap. That, too, is painful. This is one day on which you wish you had opted for a caddie or a cart. It's a painful walk back to the clubhouse.

THE FIRST DAY TREATMENT

IMMEDIATE: Stop Playing

Playing through this pain will not produce any gain. The sooner you rest the elbow and treat it, the less time it will take to heal. If you insist on playing, it's very likely the pain will eventually become so intense, and the ROM (range of motion) so limited, that for now you will have no choice but to quit.

IMMEDIATE: Ice It

As soon as possible wrap the elbow in ice for fifteen minutes. Do it a total of three times during that first day: morning, afternoon, and evening.

IMMEDIATE: Massage It

After icing, rest your extended arm on a table or desk. Massage the painful area by rubbing two fingers firmly across (up and down) the painful area for five minutes. Repeat after each icing.

RETURN TO ACTION

This will not make you happy. Plan on four to six weeks for recovery before you can return to a sport that requires the use of your elbow. Only if the pain disappears earlier and you're able to move your arm freely in all directions can you resume your game ahead of schedule.

REHAB AND PREVENTION

Rest the elbow for three days, and on the fourth day begin the R&P process.

Use a heating pad on the elbow for ten minutes before you begin the exercises. Do *not* ice it prior to exercise. During the rest of the day, *do* ice the painful area three times a day with at least an hour in between applications.

Stretching the muscles of your forearm and wrist will increase flexibility. Strengthening the muscles of your shoulder, wrist, and forearm is of paramount importance. A stronger muscle and tendon will better meet the demands of an active lifestyle.

The ROM (range of motion) exercises will increase the mobility of your elbow.

When you're at play again, wear a strap or band around your troubled forearm to alleviate excess stress. When you do return to the game of your choice, massage your elbow with ice on a regular basis after you participate.

Poor biomechanics (technique) is often the cause of medial epicondylitis. If you're participating in a sport in which you use a club, bat, or racquet, your fingers and wrist are probably in the wrong position and are not properly aligned. If you're a pitcher, your pitching motion needs work. Talk to a pro about it.

REHAB AND PREVENTION REVIEW

- ◆ Ice it!
- ◆ Heat it!
- ◆ Stretch it!
- ◆ Strengthen it!
- ◆ Strap it!
- ◆ Adjust and improve your technique!

▶ CAUTION: Use moderate heat. It's too hot if redness lasts more than one hour after heat application or if blisters form.

▶ **CAUTION:** Excessive use of ice can cause blisters or skin damage.

THE EXERCISES

Wrist stretch: 1 ◆ 2

Shoulder strengthen: 1 ◆ 2 ◆ 5 ◆ 6 ◆ 8

Elbow strengthen: 1 ◆ 2

Forearm strengthen: 1 ◆ 2

Wrist strengthen: 1 ◆ 2

Finger strengthen: 1 ◆ 2

WRIST

Carpal Tunnel Syndrome

THE PAIN

You awaken during the night and feel a tingling—pins and needles—in three fingers of one hand, most likely your thumb, index, and middle fingers. You realize the same sensation invades the area on the palm of that hand, just below the thumb. The symptoms are still bothersome in the morning, and several days later you can't quite coordinate the use of those fingers. You feel a bit clumsy as you slide a slice of bread into the toaster and lift your coffee cup. You're mystified because the feeling often disappears during the day and is not apparent when you're back in action batting a ball around. But it should tip you off that you may be suffering from **carpal tunnel syndrome.**

LOCKER ROOM LINGO

While **CTS** is the obvious shorthand, we've also heard carpal tunnel syndrome called **typist's wrist** or **jackhammer's wrist.** If you have ever operated a jackhammer, you'll know why.

THE INSIDE STORY

The carpal tunnel is an area of the wrist where tendons and the median nerve travel from your forearm to your hand. The median nerve is responsible for the feeling in your thumb, index, and middle fingers, and also their movement. If you have X-ray, or tunnel, vision, you might see that the tunnel is formed by an inflexible, leathery ligament (the

66

flexor retinaculum). There is little excess room in the tunnel, so when the tendons and nerves swell from overuse, they cause pain and tingling by increasing pressure on the median nerve.

THE RISK RATING

The pain and tingling will get worse, and the lack of coordination could become more of a problem if you don't get to work on rehabilitating it.

THE GAME

A likely scenario: You have taken up racquetball. Proudly, you adjust easily to making the swift movements and lightning decisions about where and when to address the ball. You're in good shape and you feel a surge of Glory Days excitement. You are tracking the ball with the hand and eye coordination of an expert. It's not until a few nights later, at home, that you sense you may have a problem with your racquet hand. It feels okay on the court, but not at night or in the morning. In your best superathlete terms, you announce your latest mysterious sports injury to some of your colleagues at the office. It's an ego-damaging experience when you learn your symptoms are similar to those experienced by some of your co-workers. But not your kind of people, not the athletes. Why, one of the most docile workers there, a rotund typist, says he has **carpal tunnel syndrome!** A slothful computer operator who hasn't done a lick of exercise in his life says he's a victim as well! Even your boss, whose accusing finger is the most active part of her body, has it. Must be from signing checks and dismissals! People who couldn't hit the side of a barn door with a racquet are ex-

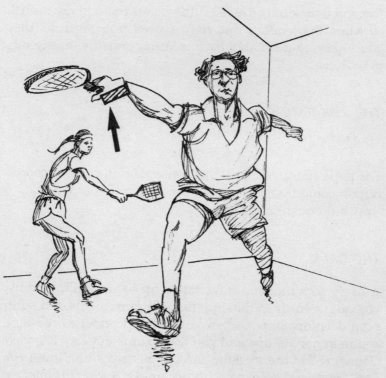

Carpal Tunnel Syndrome

pressing their sense of communion with you, the office jock! The truth is, no matter what you do, if you repeatedly hold your wrist and fingers in an incorrect way, you're at risk for developing this problem.

THE FIRST DAY TREATMENT

No need to stop playing as long as your discomfort appears to be limited to those three fingers and the thumb area. And it's not necessary to rush to the ice compartment or the medicine chest.

RETURN TO ACTION

Generally there is little threat of severe complications from continuing your regular schedule of sports activity while suffering from jackhammer's wrist.

▶ CAUTION: Don't develop tunnel vision about carpal tunnel syndrome—if the strength and coordination of your hand diminish, or if you no longer can hold a racquet or baseball bat tightly, take a conservative approach and contact your doctor.

REHAB AND PREVENTION

Keeping the wrist in a neutral position during the night usually helps relieve the problem. When you sleep, you might want to wear what is called a resting splint. If the same old pins-and-needles feeling persists after a few nights, wear the splint both night *and* day for a week. Then, begin to cut back its use gradually until you're sleeping splint free.

▶ CAUTION: Be certain the splint does not cut off circulation.

Try your ball-hitting moves in slow motion so that you can watch your wrist carefully and then possibly adjust your technique. Or ask a pro for advice on how to better hold your racquet, paddle, or bat.

REHAB AND PREVENTION REVIEW

◆ Splint!
◆ Wrist watch!

Skier's Thumb

THE PAIN

You feel a sharp pain between your thumb and index finger. It's in the area called the "web space." It's possible the sore area is swollen and black and blue. Grabbing a bat, ball, or ski pole has become a very difficult and painful experience. It even hurts to give the "thumbs-up" sign. And if you wanted to "hitch" to a ball game, you would be forced to use the other hand to "thumb" a ride. The medical term for this problem is longer than your aching thumb. It's called an **ulnar collateral ligament sprain.**

LOCKER ROOM LINGO

No matter how you suffered your sprain, it's universally called **skier's thumb.** There is also a historically correct name for it. But telling the guys that you have **gamekeeper's thumb** will sound somewhat pompous and might result in a slew of questions. So be prepared to say that the term game-keeper's thumb comes from the days before supermarkets, when gamekeepers used their hands to break the necks of small animals before sending them on their way to the dinner table. If that doesn't get their immediate respect, nothing will.

THE INSIDE STORY

One of the ligaments responsible for the stability of the thumb is the ulnar collateral. It's located in the web space between your thumb and index finger. All ligaments connect one bone to another. This one connects the hand bone (the first metacarpal) to your thumb bone (the phalanx). The ligament tears when it's stretched beyond its capacity.

THE RISK RATING

With a proper rehab program, a sprained ligament will heal. Failure to rehab risks some permanent disability, making it difficult for you to grasp things with your hand.

THE GAME

A likely scenario: You have been gliding down your favorite ski slope with remarkable ease. The lessons you took during

Skier's Thumb

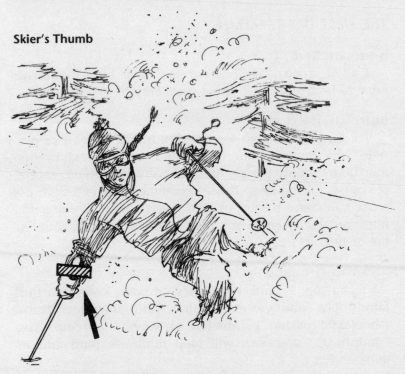

your last vacation have kicked in. You shift weight and change directions, no longer fearing you will die on every downhill run. Why, it's almost effortless. Almost. Lost in self-congratulatory thoughts of a peerless performance, you ignore the instructor's number one rule: Concentrate! Concentrate! Concentrate! A simple turn suddenly becomes a potentially traumatic event. You have skied perilously close to a treeline, edging the slope. Eyeing the trees, you lose your balance and begin to fall. Instinctively, in an attempt to regain your equilibrium, you tightly grasp one of your poles to use as a crutch. But as you fall, the force of your body weight causes your thumb to bend backwards and twist sidewards. You miss the trees, but the fall is painful to your pride, and especially to your thumb.

THE FIRST DAY TREATMENT

IMMEDIATE: **Rest**

Call it a day. You'll want to. Once hurt, ligaments have to be treated with great care. Stay by the fireplace.

IMMEDIATE: **Ice It**

Ice the painful area for fifteen minutes as soon as possible after hurting your hand. And for the next twenty-four hours repeat the ice therapy every two hours, except, of course, during sleep time. Remember that excessive use of ice can cause blisters or skin damage, and if you suffer from circulatory problems, seek medical advice about the use of heat or ice.

IMMEDIATE: **Thumbs Up**

If you can, for fifteen minutes an hour, keep your hurt hand open and elevated above your shoulder, like a schoolchild asking permission to leave the room. This "thumbs-up" approach will help minimize pain and reduce swelling.

RETURN TO ACTION

One to three weeks is the rule of thumb. In more severe cases, four to six weeks might be necessary. Do not try to test your thumb in any athletic activity until you no longer feel any pain and you can move it freely.

REHAB AND PREVENTION

Achieving your full ROM (range of motion) is necessary for the normal functioning of your hand during day-to-day activities as well as while participating in sports activities. This will require a series of easy-to-perform exercises. Strengthening your thumb and index finger will help prevent future injury.

▶ CAUTION: It's very important not to move your thumb beyond the point where it begins to feel painful.

While the injury is still painful, keep it taped or in a splint. Using strips of cloth tape, begin on the bottom of your thumb beneath the "web space." Bring the tape around and through the "web space," under your thumb, and back around in a crisscross fashion. Add strips of tape up your thumb to just below the knuckle. It's probably easier to buy a "thumb spica" splint. Worn correctly, this splint immobilizes the injured thumb in a position that promotes healing.

REHAB AND PREVENTION REVIEW

◆ ROM!
◆ Strengthen!
◆ Protect!

THE EXERCISES

Finger strengthen: 1 ◆ 2

Finger Sprain

THE PAIN

One of your knuckles is beginning to look and feel as if you have punched a brick wall. It is swollen, stiff, painful, and discolored. Making a tight fist or straightening the affected finger is difficult or impossible. It's a sure bet that you jammed your finger and have sprained a **collateral ligament**.

LOCKER ROOM LINGO

Even though it's your finger that has been injured, in some locker rooms the problem is called **coach's finger**. It's also called **jammed finger**. And we've also heard an occasional reference to **fickle finger**, as in "the fickle finger of fate has taken me out of the lineup."

THE INSIDE STORY

Each finger, except your thumb, has three joints that permit you to bend and straighten it. Any other motion that can damage your finger is restricted by collateral ligaments located on each side of these joints. These ligaments become strained when the fingers are forced to move beyond their normal range of motion.

THE RISK RATING

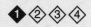

With rest your finger will get better. The ligament will heal with normal motion and function restored if you follow the rehab program.

THE GAME

A likely scenario: It's a perfect spring day. Cool and bright. The infield, to honor the new season, is raked and virtually flawless. The ball field's boundaries, straight and true, are limed pure white in what is perhaps the last clear expression in our changing society of what is fair and foul. Our eyesight may fail us, thus igniting a debate. But here, there will be no plea bargaining. It's either a hit, or it isn't. The sights and smells of the season (the outfield grass is freshly cut) and the language of the season (the upbeat chatter of your team-mates) provide sustenance to the fantasies that have long lived in your field of dreams. They tempt even the most be-

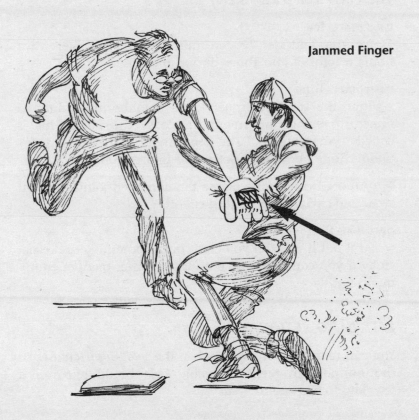

Jammed Finger

nign ballplayer to display some Sunday-morning heroics. Stepping smartly to your right, you make a deft defensive move and scoop up a hard-hit softball. It's a race now between you and the batter. A lunging last step and a creative swipe with your glove a millisecond before the runner's foot sinks into the bag produces a nifty putout. But it's impossible to accept the acclaim of your Glory Days teammates. You drop the ball, vigorously shaking your gloved hand in pain. As you brilliantly executed the play, you jammed your finger into the batter's gut. The fickle finger of fate has interrupted your season.

THE FIRST DAY TREATMENT

IMMEDIATE: **Ice**

Ice the knuckle for ten minutes. Repeat every two hours a total of four times during that day.

IMMEDIATE: **Tape**

Tape the troubled finger to its neighboring uninjured finger to restrict movement and ease the pain. This is called "buddy taping." The good finger is the bad finger's buddy. Tape above and below the injured joint.

▶ CAUTION: Do not tape across the damaged joint. It might swell and circulation could be cut off.

OPTIONAL: **Rest**

Sit it out if you feel you can't participate fully and especially if you can't grip the bat (or any other piece of equipment) tightly.

RETURN TO ACTION

You can return to your sport when the swelling decreases so that normal movement is possible. This should take from a few days to two weeks.

REHAB AND PREVENTION

Ice the finger for fifteen minutes three times a day until the swelling is almost gone. Some swelling might persist for many weeks.

Buddy-tape to limit motion and protect the joint when you first return to the sporting activity.

"Walk" your finger back to good health. This is a stretching exercise that is essential to your recovery.

REHAB AND PREVENTION REVIEW

◆ Ice!
◆ Tape!
◆ Let your fingers do the walking!

▶ CAUTION: Excessive use of ice can cause blisters or skin damage.

▶ CAUTION: If you suffer from circulatory problems, seek medical advice about the use of heat or ice.

THE EXERCISES

Finger stretch: 1

Hip Bursitis

THE PAIN

Hip pain is something you have always associated with old people. Until now. You notice that some of your simple movements are accompanied by a sharp, pinpoint pain in your hip. Little things such as walking to your car, crossing your legs while watching TV, or even sleeping on your side are painful. Occasionally the pain radiates down to your knee. The affected area might be slightly swollen and warm to the touch. The symptoms read like a case of **trochanteric bursitis.**

LOCKER ROOM LINGO

Explaining to your Glory Days chums you suffer from **trochanteric bursitis** will never sound "hip." **Hip bursitis** is the common name. **Hip burr** or **bursitis,** for short, will also do nicely.

THE INSIDE STORY

Bursitis is a problem with a fluid-filled sac called a bursa. A bursa is a part of the anatomy designed to prevent friction when muscles or tendons pass over bone. The bursa that's troubling you is located in the part of the hip called the greater trochanter. It's a natural bony bump that can be felt just below your waist. If you have a hip pocket, it's located on your trochanter. Normally, the greater trochanteric bursa is the size of a quarter, but when injured it can quickly fill with fluid and swell to as big as a golf ball.

THE RISK RATING

Rest it and there's no chance it will get worse. Without rest, your condition will just not get better.

THE GAME

A likely scenario: You almost begin to drool as the softball arcs its way down toward the center of home plate. Your perfectly timed swing sends the ball into the gap between right and center field. You feel good rounding second, intent on stretching a sure double into a triple. The third-base coach shouts "slide." Although inexperienced, you are eager to display your competitiveness. You hit the ground in a cloud of dust, sliding forward on your hip. You're safe, but not without a price. In a few days the discoloration in the hip area goes

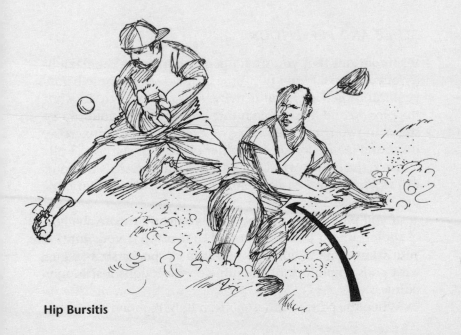

Hip Bursitis

away but not the pain. An attempt to jog it out by running a familiar route along country roads intensifies the problem.

THE FIRST DAY TREATMENT

IMMEDIATE: **Ice**

Put ice on the painful area for fifteen minutes, four times a day until the pain disappears.

IMMEDIATE: **Rest**

The hip thing to do is stay on the sidelines until the pain is gone. If you decide to play hurt, you might be forced to give it up and face a longer convalescence.

RETURN TO ACTION

Do not go back to the playing fields until you're 90 percent pain free. This could take up to six weeks.

REHAB AND PREVENTION

It's important that you strengthen and increase the flexibility of your hips. Many part-time athletes stretch only before beginning their physical activity. Our advice is to do what the pros do and help avoid future problems with your hip by stretching your muscles *before* as well as *after* you exercise. It's sound advice for keeping other muscles in shape as well.

Ice is the athlete's best friend, even when there is no pain. But when you feel susceptible, ice your hips for fifteen minutes after exercise.

If you play contact sports, or if you can't ignore the lure of sliding into a base, buy a pad that protects your hips. If your Glory Days teammates poke fun at you for showing up with pads, explain that the athlete who laughs last laughs painlessly!

When the pain is almost gone, a light regimen of jogging

is recommended. When you hit the road again, make sure it's not a hard, uneven road. Find a track or field that is firm but "gives" a bit. Also be certain the path you choose is flat. Avoid uneven surfaces, which can not only reinjure your hip but cause other problems as well.

Never play your sport in worn-out sneakers or shoes. They could be contributing to your aches and pains the way your car is affected when the tires aren't balanced or the front end is out of alignment. Save wear and tear on your hips by choosing footwear that fits correctly. While a new pair of athletic shoes might be expensive, replacing them more frequently could prove to be a bargain.

It would not be unusual for one of your legs to be slightly longer than the other. A doctor or physical therapist can quickly determine whether it's a significant and potentially injurious problem. If that is the case, a heel lift might be prescribed to even out the difference.

REHAB AND PREVENTION REVIEW

- ◆ Stretch!
- ◆ Ice!
- ◆ Pad your part!
- ◆ Jog!
- ◆ Heel lift!
- ◆ New sneakers!

▶ CAUTION: Excessive use of ice can cause blisters and skin damage.

THE EXERCISES

Hip strengthen: 1 ◆ 3 ◆ 4

Knee strengthen: 1

Hip and thigh stretch: 1 ◆ 2 ◆ 4

Iliotibial Band Friction Syndrome

THE PAIN

Every time you take a step you feel a rubbing sensation, and sometimes you may even hear a popping, snapping, or clicking in your hip or knee. It might be loud enough to become an embarrassment, so that when you and a companion go for a quiet walk or jog, the friend asks, "What's that weird clicking sound?" It's you! If this strange sensation is accompanied by pain and soreness in the hip, you're probably suffering from **iliotibial band friction syndrome.** It can be confused with bursitis, but this pain is less localized and there is no swelling.

LOCKER ROOM LINGO

Snapping hip. It not only sounds like a "hip" injury to have, it is a lot easier to pronounce. If you're a purist and disdain doing things the easy way, you pronounce "iliotibial" this way: ihl-ee-oh-tib-ee-al.

THE INSIDE STORY

The iliotibial band—the ITB—is a thick, flat, white leathery tissue that travels from the hip to just below the outer side of the knee. It travels a long way, crossing both your hip and knee joints. As it passes down across your hip, it goes over a natural bony bump called the greater trochanter. If the ITB is tight and inflexible, it stretches over the bump with difficulty and becomes very vulnerable to irritation. And as the ITB moves, a click will be felt, if not heard. However, it is stretchable, and with the rehab program can be made more flexible.

THE RISK RATING

With rest and rehab this will get better. Without rest it will be a lingering problem.

THE GAME

A likely scenario: The nature trails that snake their way through a nearby park are open to cyclists and provide a nifty way for you to build your leg muscles and stamina, and enlarge your lung capacity. During one of your outings, you become distracted by a rubbing sensation in your hip. It's annoying, but at first, it's painless. So you continue to ride your bicycle nearly every day. Soon, you realize that the rubbing sensation has given way to a "click" that occurs with every movement of your hip. You get off the bike and take a

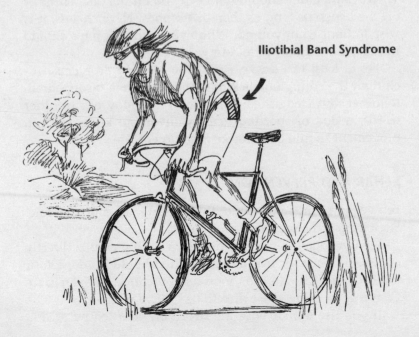

Iliotibial Band Syndrome

few steps to see if you can walk or jog it off, but the problem is apparent with every forward move you make.

THE FIRST DAY TREATMENT

IMMEDIATE: **Ice Is Nice**
Icing the area as soon as you can for fifteen minutes will help alleviate the pain.

IMMEDIATE: **Slow Is the Way to Go**
There is no need to halt your activity, but cut your pace back to minimize the stress on your ITB.

Don't be a rebel, keep it level. If the terrain ahead is very challenging, seek a more level pathway, if possible.

RETURN TO ACTION

The clicking alone should not keep you off the bike paths or on the bench as long as there is no pain. Nevertheless, it is wise to limit what you do. Whatever pain you have should not last more than two to four weeks.

For at least two weeks, even after all your problems—including the snapping/clicking/popping—have disappeared, follow a restricted schedule. A day on. A day off. In other words, a day of sporting activity involving knee and hip movement should be followed by a day off.

REHAB AND PREVENTION

You've got to make your hip, thigh, and knee more flexible. Stretching is the way to do it.

Ice-massage the affected area by rubbing a cube directly across the pain for five minutes. This should be done four times a day. Also do it as soon as you can after exercising. Continue to follow these directions for five weeks.

If you use a bike, ease the strain on your leg by raising

the height of your seat. When you pedal along, your knee should never be more than slightly bent. Follow that advice even if you feel nothing but a slight rubbing sensation in your hip or knee.

We're not interested in raising footwear sales, but it's crucial that your athletic shoes are in excellent condition. Search your sole and evaluate the wear pattern on your sneakers or shoes. If there's excessive wear on only one side of the heel, a custom-made shoe insert may be beneficial. Get the advice of a doctor or physical therapist to find out if a shoe insert is necessary for your condition.

When you run, choose the most compatible terrain. A number of painful problems related to your lower extremities (from the hip down) can be traced to running and walking on hard, uneven surfaces. Try to minimize your difficulties by being more discerning in choosing the roads, tracks, and pathways you use.

REHAB AND PREVENTION REVIEW

◆ Stretch!
◆ Ice!
◆ New shoes!
◆ Search your sole!
◆ Route cause!

▶ CAUTION: Remember that excessive use of ice can cause blisters and skin damage.

THE EXERCISES

Hip strengthen: 1 ◆ 3 ◆ 4 ◆ 5

Hip and thigh stretch: 1 ◆ 3 ◆ 4 (4 is the most important.)

THIGH

Quad Contusion

THE PAIN

The pain was an instant reminder that you had just taken a blow to your thigh. Your discomfort intensified as the thigh swelled up and likely began to turn black and blue. Quickly, it became difficult—and very painful—to bend your knee or lift your leg. You are suffering from a **quadriceps contusion**. It's a familiar problem for the Glory Days athlete who is an aggressive participant in a competitive, contact-prone sport.

LOCKER ROOM LINGO

Just simplify the terminology and all your athletic friends will know what happened to you. "I've got a **quad bruise**" is accurate and adequate. But an announcement that you "took a bad bump on the thigh" is really all you have to say to relate your bruise news.

THE INSIDE STORY

The injured quadriceps muscles travel from the hip, down the front of your thigh, over the kneecap, to just below the knee. The damage has been acute enough so that bleeding and swelling have occurred between the layers of the muscles themselves, as well as between the muscles and the leg bone (the femur), and between the muscles and the skin. Complications can develop. Sometimes in response to this kind of injury, the body develops calcium and bone in the damaged muscle fibers. The calcium and bone act like an unwelcome wedge, preventing the quad muscle fibers from interacting properly and making it extremely difficult for your knee to move naturally.

THE RISK RATING

Failure to rehab could increase the likelihood of calcium and bone deposits developing in your quad muscles, which will restrict movement of your knee.

THE GAME

A likely scenario: Your family reunion always has an athletic component. This year one of the relatives arrives with a soccer ball. Soccer is not one of your talents, but you try to re-create the moves you remember seeing on TV during the last World Cup finals. Your competitive instincts are not sub-merged for long in the familial niceties of the annual get-together. There's always an in-law who tries to show you up. You take a mental oath that it won't happen this year. But success comes with a price. You take the ball downfield with the grace of a ballerina. In full control, you feign passing off to one of your kids, to your spouse, and to your sister. In doing so, you have smartly taken the officious in-law out of the play as you head for the goal. But not for long. Your com-bative opponent is upon you, taking quick swipes at the ball, eager to trip you up in the process. It's become personal. A grudge match. And the whole family is watching! The ball bounces too high. You both go after it, legs and arms reach-ing, pumping, kicking. You artfully catch the ball perfectly with your toe. The family cheering section reacts with awe. Their shouts, however, are drowned out by your cry of pain. You've taken a knee in the thigh. And you're down. As you wince with pain you vow the offending relative is never to receive an invitation from you again. Not for the holidays,

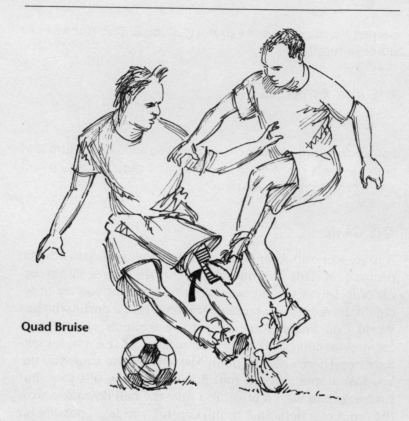

Quad Bruise

not for your kid's wedding, not for anything. But then you realize the ball actually went into the goal. You scored! So you sure will invite the relative back, so that in his presence you can recall not the pain but this moment of glory, for all the family to hear.

THE FIRST DAY TREATMENT

IMMEDIATE: **Rest**

Stop to give the thigh a rest. If it hurts only a little, and there is no swelling or discoloration, and if you can pass the following two tests, you can return to your sport after a few minutes' break.

Test One: To measure the severity of the problem, lie down. Without bending your knee, and with your thigh muscles tightened, lift your leg straight up off the ground. If you cannot tighten your thigh muscles or lift your leg without experiencing severe pain, do *not* resume your physical activity.

Test Two: If it's very painful, swollen, and discolored, do *not* return to your activity.

IMMEDIATE: **Ice**

Ice the painful area for twenty minutes. Repeat three times at two-hour intervals.

IMMEDIATE: **Stretch/Compression**

If you failed to pass either test, as soon as possible, try to bend the troubled knee past the 90-degree (right angle) point, up to 120 degrees if you can. Keep it there as often as possible for up to twenty-four hours. There are several ways of doing this:

Method 1. Usually when you sit in a chair, your knee is at the 90-degree mark. Start with your trouble side foot flat on the floor and slide it back under the chair as far as you can. Your heel might come up from the floor, but that's okay. If you need help moving that leg back toward the 120-degree position, cross your good leg over your troubled leg and slowly push it back. You will experience some pain, but it's important to stop before the pain is too much to handle. Remember to ice!

Method 2. Using a figure-eight design, wrap an elastic bandage around your thigh and knee. This will help control further swelling and discoloration, while also making it easier for you to keep your knee in a bent position.

▶ CAUTION: Keep the wrap on continuously during the day, but not while you're sleeping—you may risk cutting off your circulation, and it's possible your injury might swell up while you slumber.

RETURN TO ACTION

You should be okay to play within a week. Be certain that you can bend and straighten your troubled knee without pain. Also, perform Test One from the treatment section again. If there's no pain, you're on your way.

REHAB AND PREVENTION

When you can both straighten and bend you knee without pain, you have regained your full ROM, or range of motion. To reach that point, do some heel slides. This involves sitting on the floor or some other firm surface. Keep your back straight and your legs stretched out in front of you. Slowly slide your heel as far as you can back toward your butt. Of course, you'll have to bend your knee to do so. Then slowly return your leg, straight out, to the beginning position.

The heel slide is but one of ten EEs—essential exercises found at the end of the book—that are required to help prevent further trouble. These will not only make your thighs more supple, but strengthen them and all their support systems.

REHAB AND PREVENTION REVIEW

◆ Restore range of motion!
◆ Stretch and strengthen!

THE EXERCISES

Hip and thigh stretch: 2 ◆ 3

Knee strengthen: 1 ◆ 4

Ankle strengthen: 1

Hip strengthen: 1 ◆ 2 ◆ 3 ◆ 4 ◆ 5

Groin Strain

THE PAIN

Your inner thigh really hurts. It may bother you when you're walking along and bending down, but it's definitely painful when you squeeze your legs together. The pain is located anywhere from halfway up your thigh, to right into the groin area. You might have first felt it as a twinge that gradually increased in severity. Possibly, you were unlucky enough to have immediately suffered the full impact of the pain, as if someone tried to chisel into your inner thigh. You might have a golf ball–sized swelling in the area. If that's the way it happened and that's the way it feels, you have likely suffered an **adductor strain.**

LOCKER ROOM LINGO

If you've been horsing around, tell your paddock pals that you have **rider's strain.** We've also heard some refugees from the locker room talk about their "**GI.**" That has nothing to do with the armed forces, although it's an injury which could be caused by climbing in and out of foxholes. **GI** is short for **groin injury.**

THE INSIDE STORY

Your adductor muscles, which are strained, run from the pubic bone in your groin, down the inside of your thigh. Some end there, others continue down to just below your knee. These muscles are principally used for moving and keeping your legs together.

THE RISK RATING

If you avoid rehabbing, this injury could become a nagging, chronic problem for years to come.

THE GAME

A likely scenario: You've been doing your Dale or Roy Rogers imitation. You are so immersed in the pleasure of cantering along a woodland trail you can almost hear some campfire fiddles accompanying the Dale and Roy duet "I'm Back in the Saddle Again." You let the horse out, and it takes the hint, quickening your rush through the countryside, simultaneously quickening your heartbeat with excitement. Bending forward at the waist to avoid being bushwhacked by low-hanging trees, you tighten your thighs repeatedly, squeezing them against the belly of the sweat-glistened horse as you try to hang on. Suddenly, you feel a twinge, or a tightening along your inner thigh. Reflexively, you pull on the reins, slowing the horse so that you can gingerly dismount. Limping, you lead the horse back to its stable.

THE FIRST DAY TREATMENT

IMMEDIATE: Halt Activity

You must rest your leg as much as possible for the first twenty-four hours. The pain will likely decrease. Watch your step, and stay off stairs and hills.

IMMEDIATE: Ice

Ice the painful zone as quickly as possible. Do it for twenty minutes, and repeat every two hours during the

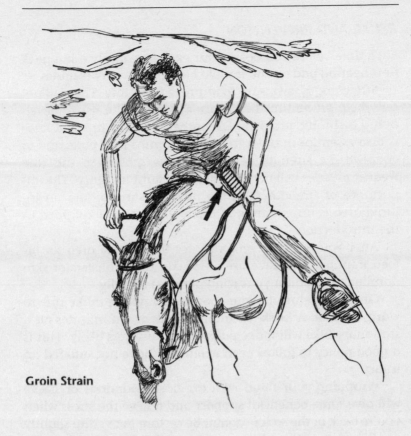

Groin Strain

waking part of the day. This will minimize the inflammation and the pain will begin to ease.

RETURN TO ACTION

When can you get back in the saddle again? Count on four to six weeks. If you're pain free sooner, you can then head for the riding trails or resume your other athletic activities. If all you feel is that "twinge" but not full-blown pain, it's wise to stop activity for the day. Try again anytime, but be vigilant. This condition could worsen.

REHAB AND PREVENTION

Each time before you begin your exercises, apply a hot pack or a heating pad on the troubled area for twenty minutes.

Stretching is necessary to improve flexibility. This will not only help prevent further injury but lessen the risk of developing a chronic problem. Strengthening your hip and knee is also essential in order to prevent strains and pulls and to equalize the strength of your muscle groups so that the weaker muscles will become more resistant to injury. The importance of strengthening the muscles surrounding an injured area is an example of linkage, which is explained in the Introduction.

After your exercise program, ice the trouble area for fifteen minutes. Excessive use of ice can cause blisters or skin damage, so monitor your icing periods carefully.

Once you return to your sporting activities, make sure to warm up first. A brisk ten-minute walk or ten minutes on a stationary bike will make pulls and strains less likely. This is a good policy to follow even when you have not suffered an injury.

Wrapping your thigh with an elastic bandage or sleeve will give some beneficial support and relieve the stress when you're back in the saddle again. Be certain to overlap slightly as you wrap while pulling up with slight pressure. Wrap the entire thigh.

▶ CAUTION: Remember that if it is too tight, the elastic bandage can cut off circulation. Do not wear it while sleeping.

REHAB AND PREVENTION REVIEW

- ◆ Heat!
- ◆ Stretch!
- ◆ Strengthen!
- ◆ Warm up!

◆ Ice!
◆ Wrap it!

▶ **CAUTION:** Use moderate heat. It's too hot if redness lasts more than one hour after heat application, or if blisters form.

▶ **CAUTION:** Excessive use of ice can cause blisters or skin damage.

THE EXERCISES

Hip and thigh stretch: 1 ◆ 2 ◆ 5

Leg stretch: 1

Hip strengthen: 1 ◆ 2 ◆ 3 ◆ 4 ◆ 5

Knee strengthen: 1

Hamstring Pull

THE PAIN

Suddenly, there is a tightening sensation in the back of your thigh. It feels as if someone has fired a walnut at you and it has lodged three inches above the back fold of your knee. Whether you attempt to run or walk, the discomfort borders on excruciating pain. Limping, however unattractive on the field of dreams, eases the pain somewhat and allows enough mobility to head toward the sidelines. You have strained your **hamstring**.

LOCKER ROOM LINGO

The Hammer! Mention it and it will attract instant attention, and sympathy, from your Glory Days peers. As in,

"What happened, my man? Did the hammer pop?" Or "Oh, no! It's the hammer! You pulled your hammer!"

THE INSIDE STORY

The **hamstring** refers to a group of three muscles located in the back of your thigh, which connects to your "butt bone" (ischial tuberosity) on one end and your knee on the other. Most often a sports injury affects only one muscle in the group. The hamstrings are used when you bend your knees and in the backward movement of your thighs. Your hamstring is activated whenever you walk or run. Hamstring injuries usually occur during acceleration, whether you're moving in a straight line or changing directions. Most "hammer" injuries are muscle strains, which are also referred to as pulls.

THE RISK RATING

If you try to play, this injury will worsen and can become a painful, long-term problem that will greatly affect your athletic performance.

THE GAME

A likely scenario: On a crisp and chilly Sunday morning, you are beckoned to a neighborhood meadow for a friendly game of football. You hear a cadence that recalls your Glory Days spent in countless huddles: "Hup one, hup two, hike!" The ball is snapped, and you move off the line and head straight down the field, confidently calling for the ball. You feel great. You arch your head upward, and there, out of the corner of your eye, is a beautiful sight. Against the backdrop of fall colors, the football spirals perfectly in your direction. Instinc-

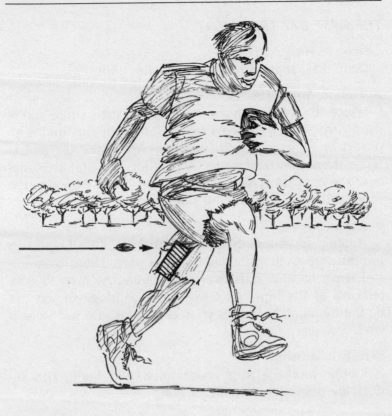

Hamstring Strain

tively raising both arms, and with fingers stretched wide, you snatch the ball from midair and smartly cradle it against your pounding chest, just like you've seen on Monday Night Football. Slightly winded, you try to accelerate toward an unmarked goal line that you have long pictured in your dreams. The touchdown that has eluded you all your life is within reach, and the fantasy is quickly becoming reality. But instead of a cry of accomplishment, you fill the air with obscenities. The pain is instant, unrelenting, and your gallop slows to a limp. It's the **hammer.**

THE FIRST DAY TREATMENT

IMMEDIATE: **Halt Activity**

Stop all activity that aggravates the pain.

IMMEDIATE: **Apply Ice**

Place the ice directly on the affected area while you're sitting up with your leg extended straight out and supported on a bench, sofa, or floor. Apply the ice for no more than twenty minutes at a time. Do it four times over the next thirty-six hours, and no more: Excessive use of ice can cause blisters and skin damage.

OPTIONAL: **Tape**

Taping or wrapping the hamstring can be helpful in minimizing swelling, but is not necessary. Use a commercial wrap or wide adhesive tape. Shave the area to ease removal of the tape. As always, the bandage should not be tight enough to cut off your circulation. Do not wear it while you sleep.

OPTIONAL: **Massage**

Gentle massage with your fingers and hands can reduce the possibility of residual pain.

RETURN TO ACTION

After thirty-six hours, if the pain has subsided, you can begin to gently stretch the hamstring. Depending on the seriousness of the strain—first, second, or third degree—it will take between two to eight weeks for your pain to disappear.

Only when your pain has disappeared should you start a more serious, yet moderate, regimen of exercises, gradually leading to a resumption of your Glory Days activities. If you can walk without pain, your next step is jogging. Jog on a flat surface! If you can jog straight ahead without pain, try cutting to the left and right. If you're still pain free, you can move to the next level and begin sprinting. Do it cautiously!

A conservative approach is important in dealing with the fickle hammer.

Ice the hammer for fifteen minutes after the first few times you return to your sport.

REHAB AND PREVENTION

Ice with a pack or bag for fifteen minutes following each exercise session.

During rehab, warm the muscles up before you do the exercises by placing a heating pad directly on the hammer for ten minutes to increase blood flow to the muscle, which will increase flexibility. Then, use a stationary bike for ten easy minutes. If you don't have a bike, take a walk on a flat surface for ten minutes at a leisurely pace.

Warm up to prevent injury when you return to your normal routines. Do light jogging, walking, or bike riding for ten minutes before engaging in your sporting activity. Stretches and strengthening exercises are essential to rehabilitating the current injury as well as preventing a repeat performance that may take longer to heal.

REHAB AND PREVENTION REVIEW

◆ Stretch!
◆ Warm up!
◆ Ice!

THE EXERCISES

Hip and thigh stretch: 1 ◆ 2 ◆ 4 ◆ 5

Leg stretch: 1

Hip strengthen: 1 ◆ 3 ◆ 4 ◆ 5

Ankle strengthen: 2

KNEE

Patellofemoral Syndrome

THE PAIN

You probably first discovered your problem as a dull soreness directly under your kneecap or possibly around the edges. It no doubt became more painful when you squatted to pick up something or climbed a staircase. That's when you likely became aware of an annoying sandpaper-like grinding sensation in your knee. Something like bone rubbing bone. It's typical of **patellofemoral syndrome** and an important difference from patella tendinitis, which is described in its own section. While there are similarities, PFS affects an area higher up than patella tendinitis, which develops in the lower portion of the knee. Another difference is the absence of swelling with PFS, and the likelihood that walking downstairs is more painful than the climb up. If you plan to watch a movie or a ball game to take your mind off the pain, forget it! The longer you sit, the more intense the discomfort.

LOCKER ROOM LINGO

Patellofemoral is either too medical or lyrical sounding to impress the sweat and muscle crowd. We suggest the simpler reference: **PFS**.

THE INSIDE STORY

Your kneecap (the patella) normally moves in a track, or groove. This problem occurs when the kneecap moves slightly outside the groove, causing the cartilage on the bottom of the kneecap to rub against cartilage on the thigh bone (the femur). Normally there is no such contact.

THE RISK RATING

If ignored, the pain will get worse and will become chronic.

THE GAME

A likely scenario: "Basic right for eight!" yelled the aerobics instructor. Her Marine drill-sergeant cadence demanded attention. "Up with the right! Up with the left! Down with the right! Down with the left!" The beat of the music, counter-

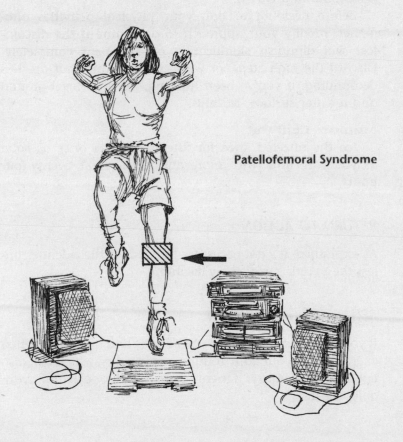

Patellofemoral Syndrome

point to the commands of the instructor, prevented you from
zoning out the way you so often did during more benign
forms of exercise. "The higher the step, the better the workout!" she exclaimed for the millionth time. It was then that
a competing message was sent from your knee to your brain:
"Something's gone wrong!" Every step up and down was
painful. And the wrong you were suffering was patellofemoral syndrome.

THE FIRST DAY TREATMENT

IMMEDIATE: **Step Down**

Before deciding to halt your physical activities altogether, modify your approach to determine if the discomfort will diminish significantly or disappear completely.
Discard the high steps, or work out on stairs that are less
demanding. If you've been running, move to level ground
and a softer surface. No hills!

IMMEDIATE: **Chill Out**

Ice the affected knee for fifteen minutes once as soon
as you can, and twice more during the next twenty-four
hours.

RETURN TO ACTION

As explained, it's not necessary to head for the sidelines unless the pain is surprisingly disabling.

REHAB AND PREVENTION

If you're predisposed to PFS, avoid hills and high steps when
exercising. In your daily routine, avoid stairs, which can also
aggravate the injury. If there's an escalator or elevator available, use it!

Do not wear worn athletic footwear. You need solid support and a cushioned sole.

After each rehab session, ice the troubled area for fifteen minutes. As a preventive measure, follow the same advice after each athletic activity, again icing for fifteen minutes.

Even when your pain disappears, use a commercially available elastic-type brace during sports activity. This will help keep your kneecap in its proper alignment.

Strengthening the knee and everything around it is good medicine. This requires the use of weights. Your goal should be to lift 15 to 20 percent of your body weight with each leg. Greater flexibility is also a goal. Follow the exercise regimen and resist the temptation to forgo these exercises.

REHAB AND PREVENTION REVIEW

◆ Stay on the level!
◆ Minimize your ups and downs!
◆ A good sole promises a happier hereafter!
◆ Chill it!
◆ Brace it!
◆ Be strong and flexible!

▶ CAUTION: Remember that excessive use of ice can cause blisters and skin damage.

THE EXERCISES

Hip and thigh stretch: 2 ◆ 3 ◆ 4

Hip strengthen: 1 ◆ 2 ◆ 3 ◆ 5

Knee strengthen: 1 ◆ 2 ◆ 3

Torn Cartilage

THE PAIN

It's as if someone is using a pair of pliers to pinch the inner part of your knee at the joint where it bends. As the pain intensifies, there may be some swelling and "locking" that create difficulty bending or straightening your knee. It's possible you sense a "clicking" in the knee joint. These are the classic signs of a **meniscal tear.**

LOCKER ROOM LINGO

We've heard it referred to as the **"t.c."** But, you might have to spell it out: **torn cartilage.** Then, if somebody still doesn't understand where and what it is, check the credibility of that person's Glory Days credentials. It's a very "popular" injury.

THE INSIDE STORY

The meniscus is a smooth-surfaced, C-shaped shock absorber that helps create a neat fit between the two bones, the femur and the tibia, that make up your knee joints. When you're on the go, the meniscus prevents the femur and tibia from scraping against each another. This cartilage, when torn, can look like a seriously frayed piece of fabric. Since there is little room for error in the knee joint, any change in the structure of the meniscus will cause discomfort. It has very little blood supply; therefore, it's very difficult for a damaged meniscus to heal itself.

THE RISK RATING

It is *not* wise to play through this pain. The potential for serious damage, if it has not already occurred, is significant.

THE GAME

A likely scenario: Using various pieces of lawn furniture, you have set up the outline of a miniature soccer field, complete with goals. Your small children are eager to take you on. You explain that a slight pain in your knee might limit your speed and range. The chatty family members accuse you of preparing an excuse for losing. You had first felt the pinching sensation during a different kind of bonding session with the children one day earlier, when you tried to teach them how to replace roof shingles on a small shed. To do so, you spent a long time on your knees, hammering nails. Since then the pain has come and gone. But as soon as the soccer match began, the problem stayed with you. The harder you played, the more intense it became. To the chant of "Chicken,

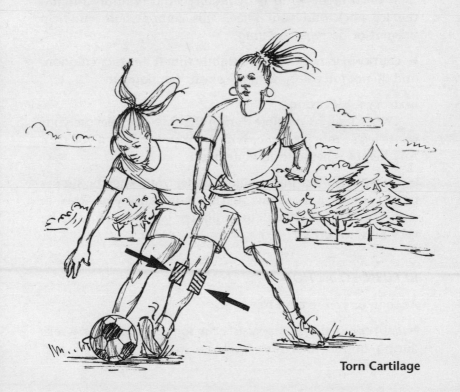

Torn Cartilage

chicken," you went to the sidelines. The player parent quickly became the coaching parent.

THE FIRST DAY TREATMENT

IMMEDIATE: **Stop**

We must stress again—it's important that you do not try to play through the pain.

IMMEDIATE: **Ice**

As soon as possible, put an ice pack on for fifteen minutes. Do it four times during the first day of pain. This will help to minimize swelling and pain.

IMMEDIATE: **Compression**

If an athletic wrap is available, wind it firmly around the ice pack and your knee. This compression will help prevent or decrease swelling.

▶ CAUTION: Do not wrap it so tightly that it limits circulation, and do not fall asleep with the elastic bandage on.

IMMEDIATE: **Elevation**

For as long as possible during the first day, elevate your entire leg so that your knee is above your hip line, if you can. Any height is better than none at all.

▶ CAUTION: Do not put a pillow under your knee or simply bend your knee to elevate it. This may cause your knee to stiffen, making it difficult to straighten your leg. This will be very hard to correct.

RETURN TO ACTION

As soon as you're pain free.

▶ CAUTION: If the pain persists for longer than four weeks during normal activities, such as walking, see a doctor.

This could be a more serious problem requiring anti-inflammatory drugs and possibly surgery.

REHAB AND PREVENTION

If any of the rehab exercises cause pain in your troubled knee, back off!

Don't be weak-kneed! It's important to keep the muscles of the legs at maximum strength and flexibility to ensure the proper mechanical functioning of your knees. Ignore the exercises at your peril. Strong legs absorb some of the stress the knees experience during normal and rigorous exercise.

After completion of your daily R&P routine, ice your troubled knee for fifteen minutes. Even when you return to the playing fields, follow this same formula to minimize the possibility of pain and swelling.

REHAB AND PREVENTION REVIEW

- ◆ Strengthen!
- ◆ Stretch!
- ◆ Limit motion!
- ◆ Ice!

▶ CAUTION: Monitor your icing carefully, as excessive use of ice can cause blisters and skin damage.

THE EXERCISES

Knee strengthen: 1 ◆ 2 ◆ 3 ◆ 4

Hip strengthen: 1 ◆ 2 ◆ 3 ◆ 4 ◆ 5

Ankle strengthen: 2

Medial Collateral Ligament Sprain

THE PAIN

There was no waiting for the agony to arrive. When you took a blow to the outer side of your knee, the pain was sharp and unrelenting. Even though your knee was banged on the outside, it's the inner side that's painful. Your knee is swollen and so stiff that it is difficult to bend. Try to bend it, and the pain intensifies. Touch the inner side of your knee, and it hurts even more. That's the classic definition of a **medial collateral ligament MCL sprain**.

▶ CAUTION: If the pain is *extreme,* and as you hobble along your knee feels as if it's about to collapse, consult a doctor immediately.

LOCKER ROOM LINGO

If you tell your Glory Days colleagues you have a **medial collateral** problem, some might think you're having trouble with a financial transaction. But the collateral here is pain. Lots of it. The locker room is more likely to understand what happened if you simply announce you have a **sprained knee**.

THE INSIDE STORY

The medial collateral ligament consists of two layers that travel from your inner thigh just above your knee, along the inner side of your leg, to just below your knee. Like a brace or hinge, the ligament is there to ensure your knee's stability when you move it from side to side or receive a bump during athletic competition.

There are three degrees of severity.

1st degree: characterized by pain but no loss of motion and minimal or no swelling.

2nd degree: swelling and more intense pain when you try to straighten or bend the knee.

3rd degree: considerable swelling, pain, and a feeling that part of your knee has become detached.

THE RISK RATING

A first- or second-degree sprain has a risk factor of 2. Failure to rehab could result in limited motion over an extended period of time. That, in turn, can result in some chronic instability or "loose knee syndrome." This is evidenced by a sensation that your knee is about to give way, or does in fact occasionally buckle.

A third-degree sprain, which is a complete rupture of the ligament, has a risk factor of 3 and a physician should be seen.

THE GAME

A likely scenario: Some people are always indifferent to the social demands of a sporting occasion. What the office bulletin board billed as a casual Sunday afternoon of touch football was marred by the overzealousness of the guys who can never seem to rein in their aggressive behavior and must prove themselves all the time, whether at work or play. But that is a psychiatric problem, you say to yourself as the game goes on. But their psychiatric problem soon becomes a medical problem for you.

Taking the ball from the center, you dash off-tackle and cut to your left, away from one of the approaching head cases. Hell-bent on roughing you up, the aggressor acceler-

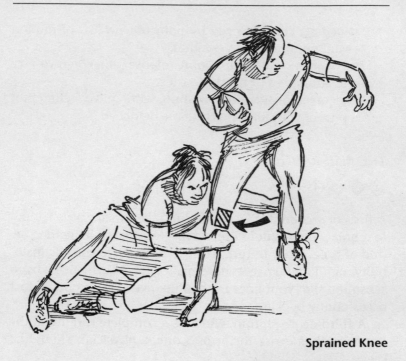

Sprained Knee

ates and soon crashes into you from the side. With the force of a hammer blow, a shoulder collides with the bone on the outer side of your knee, knocking you off balance and onto the turf. You are knee-deep in trouble. The pain is intense. You try to walk it off, but with every step you take, the added weight causes you to cry out in agony. As your co-worker expresses regret, you vow revenge. Maybe there's something you could put in the thug's Monday-morning coffee at the office.

THE FIRST DAY TREATMENT

IMMEDIATE: Stop

Stopping your activity will prevent more serious injury and will minimize pain and limit swelling.

IMMEDIATE: **Ice**

Ice the injured area for twenty minutes after the injury occurs. As you ice your knee, elevate your leg so that your knee is above your waistline. Do not bend your knee. Keep the leg straight.

IMMEDIATE: **Elevation**

Elevate your knee as often as possible during the first twenty-four hours. Again, do not bend your knee. If you work behind a desk, you have our permission to put your foot up on it. Elevating your knee will help reduce the swelling.

IMMEDIATE: **Immobilize**

While standing or walking, keep your knee straight. This will help eliminate the possibility of a permanent loss of movement or, at the very least, your being unable to completely straighten your knee.

RETURN TO ACTION

When the swelling is completely down, and you can bend and straighten your knee all the way with a minimum of pain, you can begin your rehab program. It'll take six to eight weeks after starting your rehab program before you can return to the playing fields.

REHAB AND PREVENTION

It's imperative that you are able to bend and straighten your knee soon after the injury so that you do not suffer any permanent loss of motion. So rigorously follow the exercise program listed below to ensure that you regain your full range of motion (ROM).

Strengthening the muscles of your knee and the rest of your leg will help increase stability and possibly prevent further injury. Strengthening exercises are a must. Your sense of balance must be sharpened. The balancing act is essential to help minimize the risk of unfortunate encore performances, so stick to the exercises recommended. A program of aerobic exercises will improve your conditioning and hasten the rehab process. Take your choice—bike riding, running, stepper, swimming—for twenty to thirty minutes a day.

You may need a commercially available knee brace to help keep your knee fully extended.

REHAB AND PREVENTION REVIEW

- ◆ ROM!
- ◆ Strengthen!
- ◆ Balance!
- ◆ Aerobics!

THE EXERCISES

Hip and thigh stretch: 1 ◆ 2 ◆ 3

Knee stretch: 1

Hip strengthen: 1 ◆ 2 ◆ 3 ◆ 4 ◆ 5

Knee strengthen: 1 ◆ 2 ◆ 3

Ankle strengthen: 1

Balance: 1 ◆ 2 ◆ 3

Anterior Cruciate Ligament Sprain

THE PAIN

The pain and the "pop" arrived suddenly and simultaneously. You felt or heard the "pop" as intense pain shot through the core of your knee. It likely buckled and either brought you down or made you call out for someone—or something—to keep you from falling. As the agony possibly eased somewhat, your knee has quickly swelled to the size of a grapefruit. These are the symptoms of an **anterior cruciate ligament** injury.

LOCKER ROOM LINGO

When telling your Glory Days gang about your injury, simply say **"I've blown out my knee!"** The group will understand. Around the locker room, some of your teammates might ask whether you've "torn your ACL." The painful answer is, "Yes!"

THE INSIDE STORY

The knee joint is an integral part of any forward, backward, side-to-side, or up-and-down movement of your body. The joint is formed by the convergence of the thigh bone (the femur) and one of your two leg bones (the tibia). While the knee is endowed with a lot of mobility, it does not have as much stability as other joints. There are some ligaments to help out. One of them is the ACL. It attaches to the femur at the top of the inside of the knee and travels through the joint to the bottom of the inside of the knee where it links up with the tibia. While the ACL allows the knee to do what it's supposed to do—bend and straighten—it also keeps it from popping out of position.

THE RISK RATING

There is a risk of permanent damage! Failure to rehab is certain to cause instability in your knee, possibly causing difficulty in walking but definitely limiting your ability to perform athletically.

THE GAME

A likely scenario: The temperature has just begun to drop as the sun retreats behind the glistening white slopes of your favorite mountain. There's time for just another run before the lifts close. You violate your basic rule—never to ski when you're tired. The most difficult trail of them all, the black diamond, beckons you for the first time in your brief career as a downhill skier. After all, it's late in the season, and this could be the final episode in this year's winter diary. You begin tentatively and gain confidence quickly. "What's the big deal?" you ask yourself, wishing courage had accompanied you on earlier assaults of the mountain.

The quiet of your run is interrupted by a quickening sound that is familiar to you. A snowboarder is also on a tight deadline, approaching swiftly from behind, barely in control, and about to turn the corner you have just navigated. Instinctively, you try to swing away from the center of the narrow path. As a blur of a figure passes you, your lead ski catches its tip, causing you to lose balance. You adjust, but not quickly enough. As you fall, your knee twists. You feel, and possibly hear, an ominous "pop."

You're down, screaming in pain, anger, and frustration. The sounds carry down the hill to the ski patrol, which has been waiting to survey the mountain before it's consumed by darkness. "Do you think you've blown out your knee?" the bronzed young lady in the furry orange parka asks. Her partner, examining your injury, responds for you. "Yup. It's the ACL."

THE FIRST DAY TREATMENT

IMMEDIATE: Stop

Do not attempt to play through the pain. This is one pain that will win out over any gutsy instinct to play on.

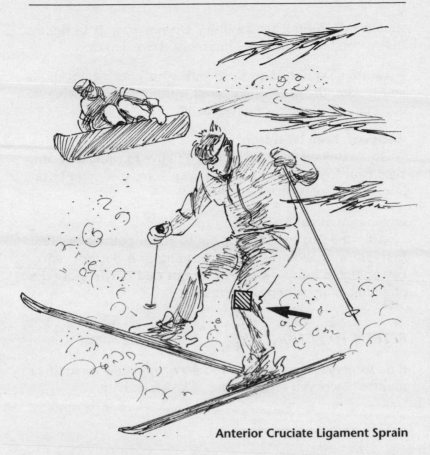

Anterior Cruciate Ligament Sprain

IMMEDIATE: **Ice It**

Wrap the knee in ice for twenty minutes. In the first twenty-four hours, do it once an hour during the entire waking day. This will minimize swelling and reduce the pain.

▶ CAUTION: Excessive use of ice can cause blisters and skin damage.

IMMEDIATE: **Wrap It**

After icing, wrap your knee with an elastic bandage. This

should help control the swelling. Do not wrap it so tightly that you cut off, or severely limit, blood circulation.

▶ CAUTION: Do not go to sleep with your knee wrapped. As you snooze, the knee might swell without your knowing it, and your circulation could be cut off.

IMMEDIATE: **Keep It Straight**
Try to stay off your leg, but if you have to walk, and can, keep your leg straight. This will keep your knee from buckling.

WARNING! **Medical Assistance**
After the first twenty-four hours, if the pain or swelling is severe, you should consider heading to a doctor's office. Potentially, a torn ACL is very serious and may require the attention of an orthopedic surgeon.

RETURN TO ACTION

If no surgery is needed, your recovery could take up to three months before you resume normal sports activity.

REHAB AND PREVENTION

Before you can start roaming the playing fields again, you must regain your full ROM (range of motion). This means when seated on a chair, you're able to hold your leg straight out without any bend in the knee. And it means being able to bend your knee fully. All, of course, without pain.

Exercising to strengthen your knee and the surrounding support systems that help keep your knee stable is essential.

Bringing a better balance to your bad leg is almost as important as bringing better balance to your life! The balance exercises help you fine-tune the movements of your knee.

Ice after each exercise session for fifteen minutes.

REHAB AND PREVENTION REVIEW

- ◆ ROM before you roam!
- ◆ Strengthen!
- ◆ The balancing act!
- ◆ Ice it!

THE EXERCISES

Knee strengthen: 1 ◆ 4

Knee stretch: 1

Hip strengthen: 1 ◆ 2 ◆ 3 ◆ 4 ◆ 5 (2, 3, 4, 5 should be done with knee and leg straight.)

Ankle strengthen: 1

Balance: 1 ◆ 2 ◆ 3

Jumper's Knee

THE PAIN

At first you sensed a slight discomfort, a soreness, just below your kneecap. Your initial reaction was typical. The pain was, you thought, an ache that would simply vanish. But the more you engaged in your favorite sports—especially those requiring a lot of jumping or squatting—the more the frequency and intensity of the pain increased. Even sitting on the bench did not prove to be helpful. The longer you sat, the more troublesome your knee became, especially when you tried to straighten your leg from the bent position. If you tried to pray for relief, and knelt on your bad knee while doing so, the pain was more acute. There's probably no swelling, unless you have been suffering from the problem for several months. Sounds like a classic case of **patella tendinitis.**

LOCKER ROOM LINGO

Please do not jump for joy when describing this injury. It'll hurt! Keep your feet squarely on the ground as you tell your buddies you have **jumper's knee.**

THE INSIDE STORY

Your damaged patella tendon connects the thigh muscles (the quadriceps) from the bottom tip of your kneecap (the patella) to the leg, where you can recognize it as the little bump on the top of your shin bone (the tibial tubercle).

THE RISK RATING

If ignored, this will become a chronic problem, so be sure to treat it immediately.

THE GAME

A likely scenario: You are a regular in the evening pickup game of volleyball. Especially proud of your graceful, balletic leaps to address the ball, you are always a leader in the scoring column. Even if the other players knew your name, they would likely refer to you by your net name, acquired through a season of airborne assaults: The Jumping Jack (or Jane). It was during an especially aggressive match that you first felt a slight discomfort in your knee. Soon, you noticed that each leap was followed by a twinge in the same knee during take-off and landing. You thought you would do the macho thing and play through the pain. But a few days later, during another match, the pain was intense enough to worry you about possibly doing some permanent damage to the knee. It was time for some treatment.

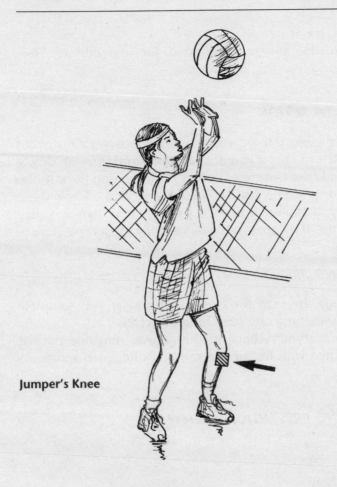

Jumper's Knee

THE FIRST DAY TREATMENT

IMMEDIATE: Come Back to Earth

Until the pain is gone, it is essential that you avoid sports activities that require you to jump, bound, or squat.

IMMEDIATE: Stair It Down

Avoid stairs whenever possible. Stairs put too much stress on the tendon that is causing the discomfort.

IMMEDIATE: **Ice It**

Ice-massage the troubled area for five minutes, five times during that first painful day.

RETURN TO ACTION

Four to six weeks is the average time for recovery. Do not cut it short. Return only if you are pain free, and start out slowly to test the knee. Example: Rather than rushing back to the tennis court, bang a few balls off a wall and address them cautiously. If you are pain free, progress to a friendly volley on the court. If all goes well, you're ready for competition.

REHAB AND PREVENTION

Ice-massage the area for five minutes after you complete your strengthening and stretching exercises.

Also, once you're back in the groove, massage the old troubled area with ice for five minutes after each sports activity.

REHAB AND PREVENTION REVIEW

- ◆ Ice!
- ◆ Stretch!
- ◆ Strengthen!

THE EXERCISES

Hip and thigh stretch: 1 ◆ 2 ◆ 3

Leg stretch: 1

Hip strengthen: 1 ◆ 2 ◆ 5

Knee strengthen: 1 ◆ 2 ◆ 3 ◆ 4

Runner's Knee

THE PAIN

There is an annoying pain on the side of your knee. It feels like a tight elastic band is slipping back and forth across the bump (the condyle) on your knee bone. An occasional "click" may be felt, or even heard. If the injury is severe, you probably are experiencing some swelling. This appears to be the knee version of **iliotibial band friction syndrome**.

LOCKER ROOM LINGO

Trying to pronounce the medical name for your problem can be risky business. If you shorthand it to **ITB** and still get blank stares in return, just tell the gang you're suffering from **runner's knee**.

THE INSIDE STORY

The iliotibial is a fibrous band that runs from the hip along the outer side of your thigh, and attaches to your leg just below the knee. You're knee-deep in trouble because the ITB has lost some of its elasticity.

THE RISK RATING

That annoying pain will become a lingering, possibly long-term problem without rehab.

THE GAME

A likely scenario: You are a creature of habit. And that habit may have caused your problem. You have long used the

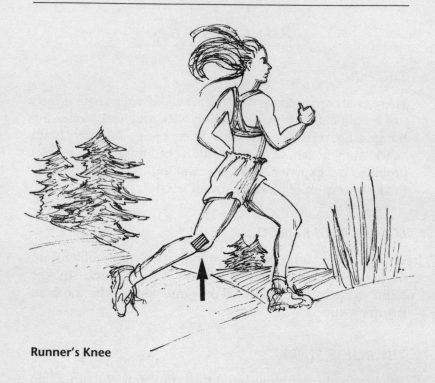

Runner's Knee

same route for your jog, either a high school track or a road that is slightly slanted or crowned in the middle. And you always run in the same direction. That means the same knee is always on the higher part of the running surface and subjected to repetitive stress. It's a sure bet that's the knee that hurts!

THE FIRST DAY TREATMENT

IMMEDIATE: Be on the Level

Choosing a level surface to run on could have an immediate effect on improving your condition.

IMMEDIATE: Slow Down

Slowing down your pace will decrease your knee's

range of motion and, in turn, should decrease the irritation on your iliotibial band.

IMMEDIATE: **Ice It**

Ice your knee for twenty minutes four times during the first day you experience the pain. Ice it as soon as possible after completing your run. Remember that excessive use of ice can cause blisters and skin damage.

RETURN TO ACTION

If you follow the Treatment directions, count on at least two weeks for the symptoms to recede. If the pain worsens or persists after two weeks, take some time off until the pain disappears.

REHAB AND PREVENTION

You have to make your hip, thigh, and knee more flexible. Stretching is the way to do it. Ignore the exercise section at your peril!

Ice-massage the affected area by rubbing an ice cube directly across the pain for five minutes. This should be done five times a day, including once soon after exercising. Follow these directions for six weeks.

It's crucial that your athletic shoes are in excellent condition so that your feet and legs are supported properly. Search your sole and evaluate the wear pattern. If there's excessive wear on only one side of the heel, a shoe insert may be beneficial. Do not use a shoe insert without the advice of a physical therapist or doctor.

Again—when you run, choose the most compatible terrain. A number of painful problems related to your lower extremities (from the hip down) can be traced to running or walking on hard, uneven or hilly surfaces. If your knee injury was caused by cycling, you can ease the strain on your leg by raising the height of your bicycle seat. When you pedal along, your knees should never be more than slightly bent.

REHAB AND PREVENTION REVIEW

- ◆ Stretch!
- ◆ Ice!
- ◆ New shoes!
- ◆ Search your sole!
- ◆ Route cause!

THE EXERCISES

Hip strengthen: 1 ◆ 3 ◆ 4 ◆ 5

Hip and thigh stretch: 1 ◆ 3 ◆ 4 (4 is the most important!)

Knee Arthritis

THE PAIN

You're convinced by now that you ought to be a weather forecaster. Your predictions are more reliable than those on your local TV station. When your knees begin to ache and stiffen, the odds are that bad weather is on its way. When that happens, your knee joints feel as if they need a lube job. The pain can be anywhere and everywhere in your knees. They feel much better when the weather is dry and cool. If they are stiff when you awaken in the morning, they'll usually ease up when you move around. While there's discoloration, some minimal swelling is not surprising. These are the symptoms of **degenerative arthritis.**

LOCKER ROOM LINGO

There's nothing very athletic about the term **arthritis.** Many jocks wince at what they believe is a synonym for old age. So among our friends, we ignore mention of arthritis and call the problem **D.J.D.,** short for **degenerative joint disease.**

THE INSIDE STORY

The smooth surface of your knee joint has, like a Cape Cod dune, been worn away by the ceaseless battering and buffeting of time, and a traumatic incident or two. There's been some loss of the knee's natural lubricant, synovial fluid. The cartilage in the joint has become bumpy, serrated, and cratered. As more of it succumbs, pain and stiffness increase.

THE RISK RATING

Arthritis will worsen. But the progression can be slowed by following the Rehab&Prevention prescription.

THE GAME

A likely scenario: It's softball Sunday and you're in bed well beyond the cranky buzz of the alarm clock, pondering the significance of a painful knee. Your thoughts scatter. You try, unsuccessfully, to reconstruct what might have caused your pain, not aware yet that the blame for this problem is the very game you've been playing for a long time. The game of life. Not aware that arthritis is the morning sickness of the aging athlete, you are psychiatrically insecure over whether it's truly your knee that is keeping you prone, or if you are subconsciously giving in to the weekly urge to skip softball and catch up on your sleep. Of course, softball wins. And during the game the pain subsides. You're happy. But not for long. The pain makes a return visit.

THE FIRST DAY TREATMENT

IMMEDIATE: Heat

Heat is the most important weapon for this injury. Use a hot pack, heating pad, or warm bath to ease the pain

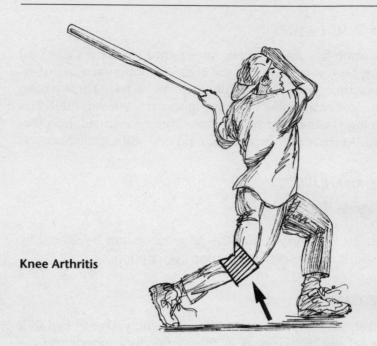

Knee Arthritis

and regain some increased range of movement. Use heat for twenty minutes, three times a day during a painful episode. We rarely recommend over-the-counter heat-producing ointments. But this is one of those times where an ointment is helpful.

IMMEDIATE: **Range of Motion**

Aid the body's natural lubricating process by *gently* moving your knee through its complete range of motion. During a flare-up, if the pain or stiffness is severe, stay off your feet as much as possible to alleviate the problem.

RETURN TO ACTION

Let your body be your guide. There's little risk in playing through the pain.

REHAB AND PREVENTION

Heat can be your best friend in treating this kind of problem. Follow the guidelines in the Treatment section above.

Remember the linkage principle. Strengthen the muscles around your knee—do not ignore any of the recommended exercises because you believe they do not *directly* relate to the knee. They do! Work on moving your knee in all its natural directions. Having full range of motion lessens the chances of knee deformities developing.

Make an impact statement by using cushioned soles. They will act as shock absorbers for every step you take. Working out on softer surfaces will also help limit the damage to your knees.

Note: Arthritis is a degenerative problem. It's possible that some of the rehab and prevention activities may, at first, make you experience more pain. But, in the longer run, you *are* helping yourself.

REHAB AND PREVENTION REVIEW

- ◆ Heat!
- ◆ ROM!
- ◆ Head for softer ground!
- ◆ Strengthen!
- ◆ Make an impact statement!

▶ CAUTION: Use moderate heat—it's too hot if redness lasts more than one hour after heat application or if blisters form.

THE EXERCISES

Hip and thigh stretch: 1 ◆ 2 ◆ 3

Hip strengthen: 1 ◆ 2 ◆ 3 ◆ 4 ◆ 5

Knee strengthen: 1 ◆ 3

Calf Strain

THE PAIN

You have a sharp pain in your calf that hurts even more when you press on it with your hand. Sometimes it feels crampy, or as if you have pulled a muscle. As you cautiously probe the painful area with your fingertips, it feels as if a large marble has been lodged there. You might notice the area is becoming black and blue. You will not want to follow anyone's advice to be "on your toes." That's when it hurts the most! You have **strained** or **pulled your calf.** Doctors use these terms interchangeably.

LOCKER ROOM LINGO

No need for a lot of bull. Simply say you've **"pulled the calf."**

THE INSIDE STORY

The calf muscles (the gastrocnemius soleus) travel from the back of the knee and leg, down to the heel by way of the Achilles tendon. The main function of this muscle group is to point the foot and toe downward for the push-off needed when walking, running, or jumping. When there's too great a load, a tear can occur in one or more of the muscles.

THE RISK RATING

Ignore rehab and this injury will become painful and will likely reoccur.

THE GAME

A likely scenario: You ran out of time and rushed to your tennis match without doing your usual warm-ups. You'll warm up by slowly getting into the game. Great theory, but it doesn't work this time. Just as you feel comfortable enough to sprint from the baseline to commandeer a ball your opponent has "wet-noodled" over the net, you are stopped in your tracks by a sharp cramping pain in the back of your calf. It really hurts! And the language you use to express that feeling as you limp to the net alerts your opponent to the fact that, for you, it's game, set, and match. You're done!

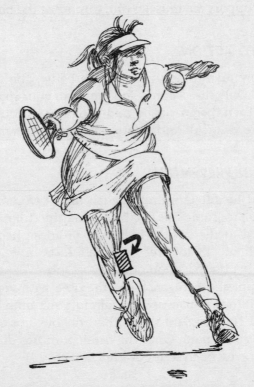

Calf Strain

THE FIRST DAY TREATMENT

IMMEDIATE: **Take a Load Off**

Immediately getting off your feet and elevating the injured leg will minimize the pain and soreness and prevent a prolonged injury.

IMMEDIATE: **Ice**

Ice the injured area for twenty minutes every four hours for a total of four times that first day of the injury.

▶ CAUTION: Remember that excessive use of ice can cause blisters and skin damage.

OPTIONAL: **Compression**

Compress the calf by winding an elastic wrap around it. That will support the muscles and minimize the pain.

RETURN TO ACTION

It will likely take three to five weeks before the symptoms disappear. Only then should you return to your sports activities. Even then, begin slowly and carefully so that you will not reinjure your calf and create a chronic problem.

REHAB AND PREVENTION

Apply heat for fifteen minutes each time before beginning your rehab program. This will help relax the calf muscle and bring blood to the area, which will promote healing. Use moderate heat. It's too hot if redness lasts more than one hour after heat application or if blisters form.

After applying heat, massage the area with your fingers for five minutes. Move upward along your muscle toward your knee. The pressure should be firm but not enough to cause additional pain. Once the acute pain has diminished, begin your prescribed series of stretches.

Strengthening exercises to firm up your calf muscles and the rest of your leg are essential to ensure you'll be able to meet the future demands of your favorite sports activities. During the rehab period, when you're not exercising, it's wise to give your calf muscles a rest. Walk in a flat-footed manner, not getting up on your toes.

Also, during the rehab period, put a lift (just a ¼-inch-thick piece of felt will do) in your trouble-side shoe.

With all calf injuries it's especially important to stretch and warm up before you begin your sports activity.

REHAB AND PREVENTION REVIEW

◆ Heat!
◆ Massage!
◆ Stretch!
◆ Strengthen!
◆ Give it a lift!

THE EXERCISES

Hip and thigh stretch: 1

Leg stretch: 1 ◆ 2

Ankle strengthen: 1

Shin Splints

THE PAIN

Every step you take is painful, whether you're running, jogging, or simply walking. The pain is also generated if you stretch your ankle by pointing your toes down. You feel the discomfort beginning just below your knee, and either down the front of your leg or down the big-toe side of your leg. Stop moving, and the pain stops. Resume your activity, and the pain returns. It can be most painful when you take your first steps out of bed in the morning. Curiously, it can be very intense when you begin your exercise program or sports activity, and perhaps eases up the more you do. Welcome to **medial tibial stress syndrome.**

LOCKER ROOM LINGO

If there were a rap group called the "Orthopedic Surgeons," the phrase **"medial tibial"** might be perfect as a repetitious rhythmic phrase. But until such a group exists, use a familiar old expression when you describe your injury to the Glory Days gang—**shin splints!**

THE INSIDE STORY

The tibia in "medial tibial syndrome" is, of course, the leg bone. Shin splints can be the result of several problems. The membrane (the periostum) that surrounds the leg bone may be pulling away from it. The membrane might also be inflamed from overuse. Or possibly the muscles in front of the leg have suffered a tear. It's impossible to distinguish one from the other. The pain, as well as the treatment, is the same.

THE RISK RATING

This injury can grow progressively worse. Without proper care you'll suffer more often and the pain will be more severe.

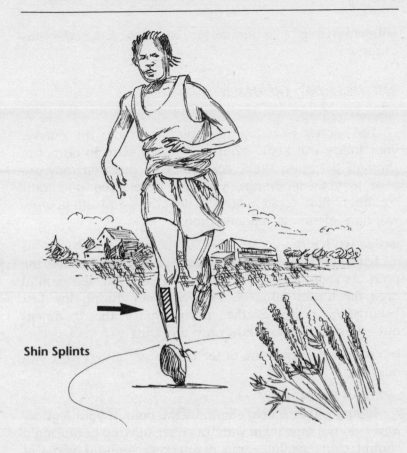

Shin Splints

THE GAME

A likely scenario: As one of the diehard runners left over from the running boom of the '70s, you religiously go out for your daily run. Bored with the routine you have established for yourself, you decide to give up running on the local high school's soft dirt outdoor track and take your act "on the road." The change in scenery is refreshing, but the change in running surfaces proves to be damaging. During the first week of using the new route, you begin to feel a strong pain in one of your legs. Most frequently, the pain develops when going from a soft to a hard surface rather than the other way around.

THE FIRST DAY TREATMENT

IMMEDIATE: Stop

The sooner you stop the painful activity the quicker your injury will heal. What you do *not* want to do is run through the pain. While continuing to push on may appeal to your self-image, you risk developing a chronic condition that could require a lengthy—and often unrewarding—period of rehabilitation.

IMMEDIATE: Ice It

Icing it will reduce the inflammation and decrease the pain. As soon as possible, get an ice bag onto the painful area for fifteen minutes. Ice five times during the first twenty-four hours of the injury. Space the treatment out—do not ice more than once an hour.

▶ CAUTION: Excessive use of ice can cause blisters and skin damage.

OPTIONAL: Tape It

Taping will also help eliminate the pain. If your legs are hairy, do not tape them without either shaving or placing a commercially available underwrap on the painful area. Cut the tape into eight-inch strips. Tape from two inches above the injury to two inches below. Begin the taping on one side of your leg, going behind your leg and around the front, in a crisscross pattern.

▶ CAUTION: Do not wrap so tightly that you cut off circulation.

RETURN TO ACTION

When you are *completely* pain free you can resume your athletic activities. The pain will likely be gone within two weeks if this is the first, or just an occasional, episode of shin splints. However, a chronic condition could keep you sidelined for several months. Ease into your running regimen. Be certain your athletic shoes are in good shape and stay on softer surfaces—grass or dirt—and only gradually return to harder surfaces if that's where you want to run.

REHAB AND PREVENTION

Poor ankle alignment and worn-out footwear are major causes of shin splints. Don't wear worn-out athletic shoes. Be certain they fit well and firmly support your feet. Again, do some research and carefully examine your shoes. A shoe that provides additional shock-absorbing capability may help reduce your susceptibility to shin splints. If you notice that your athletic shoes show excessive wear in just one spot, or they always wear out quickly in one particular area, pay attention! The shoe may be telling you that your ankle alignment is poor or weak.

The road to pain-free shins is not toll free. It includes regular trips to the exercise section of this book. Build up strength in your ankles and the rest of your legs. By making them stronger you'll take off some of the pressure on the shin itself. Work on providing freer movement for your thighs, hips, and calves. Stretching them not only gives you additional mobility but helps you perform with more precision. As is the case with just about any mode of transportation, proper wheel alignment is necessary for trouble-free movement. So it is with your "wheels." The stretches will help your front-end alignment.

When you "step out" again, be certain to do so on the best surface for you. You're likely to find your legs ache less on some surfaces than others.

If your problem persists, consider using a custom-designed shoe insert as part of the R&P process.

Each day when you've completed the total package of R&P

activities, chill down the troubled area. A five-minute ice massage is all you need. An ice massage should also be part of the end routine once you have resumed running.

Crosstraining—participating in a lower impact activity—will help you maintain your fitness level. Cycling and swimming are great alternatives. Because of your shin splint problem, when you cycle, place your foot flat on the pedal.

REHAB AND PREVENTION REVIEW

- ◆ Ice!
- ◆ Surface change!
- ◆ Shoe check!
- ◆ Step check!
- ◆ Strengthen!
- ◆ Stretch!
- ◆ Crosstrain!

THE EXERCISES

Ankle strengthen: 1 ◆ 2 ◆ 3 ◆ 4

Hip strengthen: 1 ◆ 3

Leg stretch: 3

Hip and thigh stretch: 1 ◆ 2

Achilles Tendinitis

THE PAIN

There is an annoying soreness or "twinge" in the back of your leg, one or two inches above and behind your ankle. It's as if a tight piece of fabric or leather in there is about to tear. You feel it not only when you run but also when you walk. And it's sometimes matched by a burning pain in the same area when you get out of bed after a restful night's sleep. As an active athletic person, you have shrugged off a wide variety of minor aches and pains as the price of being a jock. But this persistent soreness is forcing you to take notice. It's a safe bet that you're suffering from **Achilles tendinitis.**

LOCKER ROOM LINGO

The **Achilles!** It is a name born in Greek mythology. Achilles is the heroic figure of Homer's *Iliad*, a superhero whose fatal weakness was in his heel. You've probably used the term "Achilles' heel" as a clichéd reference to a destructive flaw in someone's body or psyche. Indeed, if you do not respond properly to Achilles tendinitis, the result, while not deadly, could be "fatal" to your Glory Days ambitions. You must take care of your Achilles or your Achilles just might take care of you!

THE INSIDE STORY

The Achilles tendon connects the calf muscle to the heel and helps to point your foot downward. The motion is necessary for walking, running, and jumping.

The Achilles tendon, and the structure surrounding it—the paratenon—are elastic-like and have probably been called upon to perform activities for which they are neither strong nor flexible enough. The result is an inflammation and quite likely one or more microscopic tears.

THE RISK RATING

If not rehabilitated properly, this could lead to a tendon tear! Tear the tendon and you have a much bigger problem, including long-term disability and pain.

THE GAME

A likely scenario: For a moment your driveway is the Boston Garden of your dreams. You're going one-on-one with your son. You reach into your memory bank for a clever stutter step that surprises him. He commits toward the hoop. You pull up quickly for a jump shot and the ball swishes through the net. But the prideful moment is spoiled. You felt a twinge in the Achilles area when you went up for the shot. As the game goes on, the soreness returns whenever you jump for a rebound and even when you go up on your toes. One of your body's shock absorbers has been injured. The **Achilles tendon** fits that description.

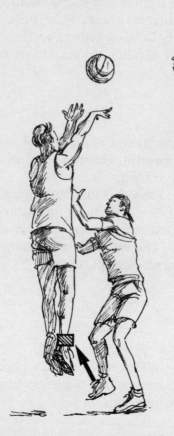

Achilles Tendinitis

THE FIRST DAY TREATMENT

IMMEDIATE: **Ice**

Put an ice pack on the affected area and keep it there for ten minutes. Repeat three times a day.

▶ CAUTION: Monitor your icing, as too much can cause blisters and skin damage.

IMMEDIATE: **Rest**

It's okay to gingerly walk on the gimpy leg if pain allows. Avoid stairs and definitely do not head back into the game. If stairs are unavoidable remember this: "Good foot to heaven, bad foot to hell." In other words, when walking upstairs lead with your good foot, then place your bad foot on the same stair. When walking downstairs, reverse the process by leading with your bad foot.

OPTIONAL: **Heel Lift**

Placing a heel lift in your shoe can ease the tension on your tendon. Lifts can be purchased, or made at home by cutting a heel-sized quarter-inch-thick pad of felt.

▶ WARNING! If you felt a **pop** in the back of your leg when you suffered the injury and could not get up on your toes, go to an emergency room or your doctor immediately. It could be a rupture, which is much more serious than tendinitis.

RETURN TO ACTION

If you're lucky, the recuperation may take only several days, although a period of weeks could be required even if a chronic condition does not develop.

It's okay to perform the ADLs (the activities of daily living), including a moderate amount of walking. But stay away from more physically challenging activities until you can get up on your toes without feeling any pain.

REHAB AND PREVENTION

If the pain intensifies during the recuperation period, or there is no improvement within two weeks after the injury is first felt, consult a physician.

Only when you no longer feel any pain or stiffness should you begin a program of gentle stretching and strengthening exercises. Improve flexibility and strengthen the Achilles before resuming a very light running regimen.

Massage the tendon with ice after each run, or other athletic event, to help prevent the Achilles from becoming inflamed again. Rub an ice cube directly across (side to side) the painful area, not up and down. Do so for five minutes just once, *as soon as possible* after you have exercised. Follow this ice massage "prescription" for three months.

If the heel lift has helped you in the hours immediately following the injury, you might find it will provide continuous benefits during sports activity. If your condition worsens, try the heel lift, even while you're doing the ADLs.

▶ CAUTION: An Achilles problem unattended will often develop into chronic tendinitis. The pain becomes more intense and widespread, and can be felt not only while walking upstairs but even on level ground. This phase is often accompanied by swelling behind the ankle. It's now even more imperative to rest the tendon, meaning no climbing, jumping, or walking. Again—icing is essential!

REHAB AND PREVENTION REVIEW

◆ Stretch!
◆ Strengthen!
◆ Ice!
◆ Keep a heel lift handy!

THE EXERCISES

Leg stretch: 1 ◆ 2

Hip and thigh stretch: 1

Ankle strengthen: 1

Achilles Tendon Rupture

THE PAIN

It initially felt as if you had been shot, stabbed, or kicked by a mule in the back of your leg just above the ankle. Reflexively reaching around to grab the painful area, you were shocked to feel a lump, which had quickly grown bigger than a golf ball. In an effort to relieve the pain, you try to point your foot downward, but you can't! An attempt to stand on your toes also fails! You can walk, but with great difficulty and a pronounced limp. You're suffering from a **ruptured Achilles tendon.**

LOCKER ROOM LINGO

Achilles was a figure in classic Greek literature whose weakness was in his heel. His flaw was fatal, and as an active person for whom sport is a metaphor for life, you will not be blamed for feeling that you too have suffered a mortal blow. So, when asked about your injury, just say **"Achilles."** And limp away.

THE INSIDE STORY

As with all tendons, the Achilles connects the calf muscle (the gastrocnemius) to the heel bone (the calcaneus). It is part of a remarkable transportation system that allows you to "push off" after receiving a message from your brain to walk, run, or jump. In this case the tendon has torn apart and is in two pieces.

THE RISK RATING

Get the phone number of a top-notch orthopedic expert and dial it without delay. Prepare to hear the words surgery or brace, or both.

THE GAME

A likely scenario: You were feeling great! No aches. No pains. Not the slightest hint of trouble on the way. So, with the crack of the bat you raced to first base, and urged on by the shouts of teammates, increased your momentum trying to stretch a solid single into a dubious double. You never made it. Your Achilles, which easily handled the elastic-like give-and-take of your run to first, snapped as you increased your stride for the gallop toward the base ahead. Down you went. Writhing in agony, you reacted with an uncharacteristic volley of ob-

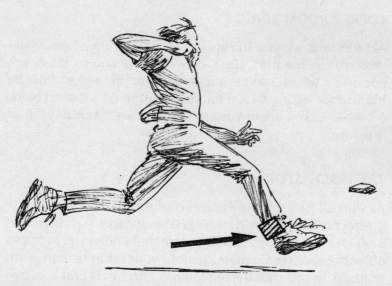

Ruptured Achilles Tendon

scenities as several of your less informed athletic friends suggested "walking it off" and trying to play through the pain. Something you would not be able to do!

THE FIRST DAY TREATMENT

IMMEDIATE: **Halt Activity**

If for some medically unexplainable reason this injury did not force you to the sidelines, that's where you belong! Get off your feet and stay off!

IMMEDIATE: **Ice**

Quickly wrap your injured ankle in ice for twenty minutes. Then take a break for twenty minutes. Repeat the process as often as possible during the first day: twenty minutes ice on, twenty minutes ice off.

▶ CAUTION: Don't overdo the ice, as it can cause blisters and skin damage.

IMMEDIATE: **Elevation**

Keep your foot elevated. When sitting, put it on a chair in front of you. When lying down, keep it as high as possible. This will help reduce pain and swelling.

IMMEDIATE: **Compression**

Keep the ankle in an elastic-type wrap, but keep it loose enough so any further swelling will not cut off your blood circulation. A circulation interruption is a big risk with catastrophic ramifications.

▶ CAUTION: Be alert. Do not wrap tightly, and do not fall asleep with the wrap on.

RETURN TO ACTION

Unless you have extraordinary recuperative powers, count on being out of action for four to six months. No typo here— four to six *months!*

REHAB AND PREVENTION

Once an MD assumes control of this injury, you likely will be given a rehab program that relates to the kind of treatment you have received.

There's no doubt that by properly warming up and increasing the strength and flexibility of your leg, you will hasten your comeback and lessen the likelihood of reinjury.

REHAB AND PREVENTION REVIEW

- ◆ Warm up!
- ◆ Flexibility!
- ◆ Increased strength!

THE EXERCISES

Hip strengthen: 1 ◆ 3 ◆ 4

Knee strengthen: 1 ◆ 2

Ankle strengthen: 1 ◆ 2 ◆ 3 ◆ 4

Leg stretch: 1 ◆ 2

ANKLE

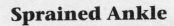

Sprained Ankle

THE PAIN

Is it just a minor twist or is it a **sprained ankle?** If it's painful when you walk, tender when touched, and swollen on the outside and front, there's little doubt it's a sprain! That diagnosis will be ratified a few hours later if the ankle turns black and blue. Try to walk and you'll get a more painful indication of what has happened. When you take the pressure off the foot and let it dangle, you'll probably feel a throbbing sensation. Over the next twenty-four to thirty-six hours it's likely to get worse—more swollen and more painful—before it gets better!

LOCKER ROOM LINGO

There is no glamorous name for **sprained ankle!** Declare that your "ankle is sprained" and your Glory Days colleagues will wince, understanding your pain. Ankle sprains are regular visitors to playing fields and locker rooms the world over.

THE INSIDE STORY

The ankle is endowed with a wide range of motion to adapt to changes in surfaces. As the ankle performs, it is stabilized by cordlike ligaments located on all sides, connecting down to the foot. A sprain usually involves the anterior talofibular ligament, which is located on the outside front of the ankle. An extreme turning of the ankle causes the ligament to be stretched beyond its normal ability. While the ligament never returns to its original length, there is a natural healing

145

process that provides some stability. However, maximum stability can be achieved by following the rehab program.

THE RISK RATING

The pain and swelling can eventually go away on their own. But without rehab an unstable ankle may result, causing recurring sprains.

THE GAME

A likely scenario: The ball arcs toward the hoop and you try to position yourself for a possible rebound. Your eye is fixated on the ball. Your movements are automatic. You snatch the ball in midair as it caroms off the rim. It's always a good feeling no matter how often you've done it. Before your feet even touch the floor, you're celebrating another successful rebounding effort and are already calculating what it will take to get the ball downcourt. But, an inadvertent bump from behind pushes you off balance slightly and within a millisecond, everything has changed. You land on the outer edge of your foot. The pain is excruciating. The ball rolls free as you drop to the floor. Time out! The words "**sprained ankle**" are repeated like a mantra from the sweat-stained Glory Days bunch who prayerfully, it seems, are trying to excise any such condition from their future lives.

THE FIRST DAY TREATMENT

IMMEDIATE: Get Off Your Feet

Sometimes you'll see a professional athlete return to the game after suffering a sprained ankle. It's likely the team's trainer has sprayed it with a deep, penetrating painkiller and provided first-rate emergency treatment in

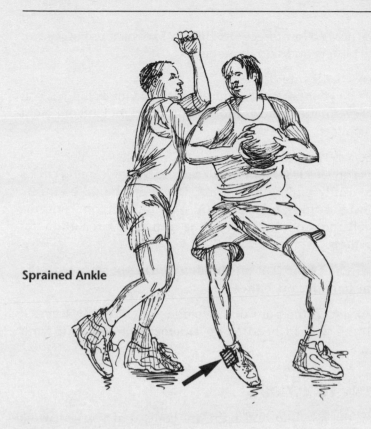

Sprained Ankle

the locker room. Hobbling back on the court, the player is applauded for an act of bravery. However, it's not advisable for you to do so! Unlike the pro, you're not playing for money and you risk a lasting injury. Stay off your foot. You'll probably have little trouble convincing yourself to remain immobile because any movement of a severely sprained ankle can generate shock waves of pain.

IMMEDIATE: **Ice**

Quickly pack the entire affected area in ice for fifteen minutes. Repeat this procedure as often as possible on that first day: ice pack on for fifteen minutes, ice pack off for the same length of time.

▶ CAUTION: Follow directions closely. Excessive use of ice can cause blisters and skin damage.

IMMEDIATE: **Elevate It**

Lie on your back with your leg elevated for as long as you can. Several firm pillows provide just the right kind of height and comfort.

IMMEDIATE: **Wrap It**

Use an elastic wrap. Wind it around in overlapping circles while gently pulling it upward. The wrap should be firmly against the ankle, but be careful. Your ankle might continue to swell and result in the bandage cutting off circulation if it is too tight.

▶ CAUTION: Do not cut off circulation. Do not sleep with the elastic bandage on, either.

▶ WARNING! If the pain and swelling are extremely severe it might be wise to head to an emergency room or to your doctor.

RETURN TO ACTION

When the swelling and pain are gone, and you can walk firmly without a limp, it's time to "ease" back into your old athletic routine. Do so while wearing an ankle support that really gives support! High-top sneakers can help, but often do not do the job. If you think you're about ready to go full tilt, you might want to wear a commercially available splint or brace, such as an air cast, for additional support.

The degree of your sprain will determine how much time you will need to sit out. A first-degree sprain (the least severe, characterized by pain but with minimal or no swelling or disruption of the muscle or ligament fibers) should take a few days to a week to heal. Second-degree sprains (moderate disruption of the fibers, increased pain and swelling along with some bruising) will take two to four weeks. Third-degree sprains (a complete tearing or rupture of the ligament or muscle fibers with maximal swelling and bruising, as well as a feeling of instability and weakness in the ankle) will take up to four to six weeks to heal.

REHAB AND PREVENTION

Strengthen your ankles and the surrounding support systems.

Work on bettering your balance so when you walk or run your foot hits the ground properly. To compensate for lost support, it's imperative to perform strengthening exercises for the other support systems of the ankle.

To guard against future sprains, always wear the proper footwear. Replace when they no longer provide firm support or adequate cushioning.

REHAB AND PREVENTION REVIEW

- ◆ Exercise!
- ◆ Perform a balancing act!
- ◆ Change your shoes!

THE EXERCISES

Hip strengthen: 1 ◆ 3

Ankle strengthen: 1 ◆ 2 ◆ 3 ◆ 4

Hip and thigh stretch: 1

Leg stretch: 1 ◆ 2

Balance: 1 ◆ 2 ◆ 3

Plantar Fasciitis

THE PAIN

Every time your foot hits the ground it feels as if you're landing on hot coals or tacks. It's a strange sensation usually located along the inside edge of the sole of your foot, just in
front of your heel. You find that, unlike most sports-related
pain you've experienced, these symptoms bother you mostly
when you're resting or getting warmed up, not while you're
exercising. Often the pain diminishes during a spirited workout and returns afterward. You're probably suffering from a
problem that sounds as strange as it feels: **plantar fasciitis.**

LOCKER ROOM LINGO

Because it can feel as if someone is playing a practical joke
by giving you a hot foot, some amateur jocks we know refer
to plantar fasciitis as **hot foot.** And, as is the case with that
other kind of hot foot, if this one is initially ignored, the problem will grow progressively worse.

THE INSIDE STORY

The bottom of the foot contains many structures that work
in sync for normal walking and running. The plantar fascia
is one of them. Thick and leathery, it connects from your heel
to the ball of your foot and assists in maintaining the arch
of your foot. When you walk or run, you go from a low-arch
to a high-arch position. When the plantar fascia has been
repeatedly stretched beyond its normal limit, it becomes
inflamed and microtears can occur. Part of the irony of this

150

injury is that the pain eases if you play through it, but returns when you have stopped. It's not that much of a mystery, though. By continuing to play, you warm up the troubled area, resulting in increased flexibility and blood flow to the fascia, which in turn decreases pain. The pain then returns because the fascia cools off.

THE RISK RATING

If you don't cool this hot foot the pain will become a chronic one, requiring more time away from your favorite sport. So, get into the rehab habit.

THE GAME

A likely scenario: From the moment you awaken in the morning and walk the dog the sole of your foot is sending messages. Something is wrong! But there is a big volleyball match on your schedule that night. Frustrated by the pain's persistence throughout the day, you decide to see if you can play through it. Your first few movements are not very encouraging. It's as if you're running on a carpet of hot coals. After you leap into the air to crunch the ball over the net, you feel as if you've landed on a bed of nails. You consider calling in a replacement and moving to the sidelines but decide to give it another couple of minutes. As the match continues, you realize the pain in the sole of your foot is becoming less intense and almost disappears. Aha! You're elated! You have experienced a Glory Days epiphany! You have played through and defeated the pain. However, the mood is soon devoured by agony. Within minutes of saying your high-five good-byes to your teammates, there again is that notorious feeling in the bottom of your foot. It is the scourge of **plantar fasciitis.**

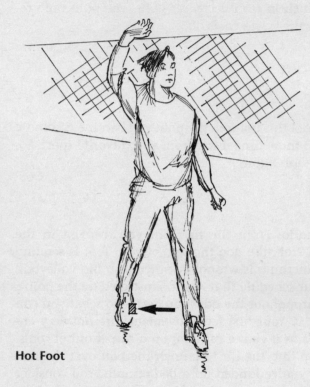

Hot Foot

THE FIRST DAY TREATMENT

IMMEDIATE: Rest

Complete rest of the painful area is the most important component of treatment. Do not participate in any activity that can aggravate the condition.

IMMEDIATE: Ice

Ice should be used as a massage three times a day. Gently rub an ice cube across the painful area for five to ten minutes. This should be done until all symptoms are gone.

▶ CAUTION: Remember that excessive use of ice can cause blisters and skin damage.

▶ CAUTION: If you suffer from circulatory problems, you should seek medical advice about the use of heat or ice.

RETURN TO ACTION

Don't test your foot in competition until you're certain it no longer bothers you during ordinary day-to-day activities. That happy juncture could arrive in just a week. However, it's not unusual for the symptoms to hang around for several weeks longer.

REHAB AND PREVENTION

Once the symptoms are completely gone it's important to begin a program of gently stretching the muscles in the back of your affected leg and bottom of your foot. The recommended stretching exercises for your ankle, hip, and calf are important because one of the main culprits causing this condition is tightness in the Achilles tendon and your calf muscles.

If flat feet are responsible for the problem, a custom-made orthotic shoe insert may help by keeping the arch of the foot elevated. You might try a heel lift to raise it by a quarter of an inch to minimize stress.

REHAB AND PREVENTION REVIEW

◆ Stretching!
◆ Special shoe insert!
◆ Heel lift!

THE EXERCISES

Ankle strengthen: 1 ◆ 2 ◆ 3 ◆ 4

Foot strengthen: 1

Hip and thigh stretch: 1

Leg stretch: 1 ◆ 2

Turf Toe

THE PAIN

Your big toe hurts whenever you put weight on it! Your instinct is to follow a coach's admonitions, telling you to be tough and "toe the line," but you still hold back, or at least automatically grimace from the expected soreness. The pain, which is likely to intensify after the first twenty-four hours, is centered underneath your swollen toe, probably enough for your shoe to feel too tight. The toe is probably turning black and blue where it meets your foot. You are suffering from a **hyperextension** injury to your big toe.

LOCKER ROOM LINGO

Turf toe! It's a most appropriate name, because this injury came into prominence when artificial turf became the choice surface on many of America's playing fields.

THE INSIDE STORY

The joint of your big toe is surrounded by tendons, ligaments, and a sheath of soft tissue. This tissue helps provide nutrition and stability to the joint of the toe. When the joint is pushed beyond its normal range, the sheath is torn.

THE RISK RATING

①② ❸ ④

There is potential for more trouble than you might think. You can become disabled by losing mobility in your toe. Persistent pain can result.

THE GAME

A likely scenario: You and your Glory Days buddies are gung-ho about receiving permission to play your weekend touch football game on the artificial turf of a nearby junior college. As you confidently sprint onto the field, you are almost daz-

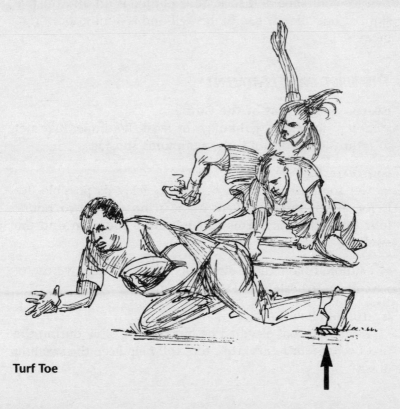

Turf Toe

zled by the undeviating bright green carpet underneath your feet. The factory-installed white yard markers, almost monotonously perfect in width and color, lend a video-game sense of visual unreality to the afternoon. It's very noticeable that this synthetic surface is demandingly different on your legs from the feet up. With the game under way, you leap to snatch a wobbly spiral and then plant your feet firmly so that you can perform a showy maneuver to elude the fast-approaching defender. But your bodies collide. With your foot still flat on the ground, you fall forward, causing your big toe to be forced backward. The pain is sudden and sharp. For a moment you think you have broken your toe. The game is stopped and you are the center of attention as you remove your shoe and sock. Your big toe is an unattractive sight. It has already begun to swell and is almost too stiff to bend.

THE FIRST DAY TREATMENT

IMMEDIATE: Stay Out of the Game

You're finished for the day, at least. It's imperative not to return to action until the symptoms subside.

IMMEDIATE: Ice

Get some ice onto the ache as quickly as possible. Ice it for fifteen minutes. Repeat the icing every two hours, four times that day. This will minimize the pain and the swelling.

▶ CAUTION: Follow these directions closely—excessive use of ice can cause blisters and skin damage.

IMMEDIATE: Elevation

Keep your foot elevated as much as possible during the first twenty-four hours. This, too, will help keep the swelling down.

RETURN TO ACTION

Any sport that puts pressure on your troubled toe should be avoided until you are pain free and can move your big toe around without difficulty. Plan on one to four weeks of down time.

▶ CAUTION: A return to action too soon will likely prolong this injury and cause permanent stiffness.

REHAB AND PREVENTION

Attaining full range of motion is mandatory to prevent further injury to your big toe. But first, it has to heal. As long as there is pain, swelling, or discoloration, ice the injury two times a day, morning and evening.

To heal, the toe must be taped in a straightened position to limit motion. Use strips of tape five inches long. Start with the first strip of tape on top where your toe meets your foot. Bring the tape down under your toe and crisscross it back up to the starting point. Move each strip forward a bit so that you have a chevron effect.

▶ CAUTION: Remember that taping too tightly can cut off circulation.

When the pain has subsided, there are two ROM maneuvers you should execute. With your hand, gently push your toe backward until you feel a stretch on the bottom of the foot and toe. Hold for one second, then release. Gently bend your troubled toe forward until you feel a stretch on the top of your foot and toe. Again, hold for one second, then release. Do this exercise, alternating between backward and forward motions, a total of ten times in each direction. Do that three times a day, every day, until you can move your toe in a normal way.

More than a stiff upper lip, a stiff lower sole can be important in resolving a turf toe problem. While you're still being bothered by turf toe, wear the stiffest pair of shoes you own for walking. For sports in which you can get bumped around, keep your turf shoes in the closet and wear the stiffest sneakers you can find. To further stiffen and limit flexibility of the athletic shoe on your bad foot, you can add an extra inner sole. Flexible steel inner soles are also available.

While newly designed turf shoes help athletes to get a better grip on things, the flexible footwear can fail to provide a strong "envelope" in which toes are protected from awkward bends and twists.

REHAB AND PREVENTION REVIEW

◆ ROM!
◆ Ice!
◆ Tape!
◆ O Sole Mio!

THE EXERCISES

Foot strengthen: 1

SKIN

<u>Chafing</u>

THE PAIN

You feel a stinging or burning sensation in your armpits or between your thighs. The more the sweat pours out of you, the more pain you feel. When you shower, the pain becomes even more intense. Lifting your arm, or peering between your legs, you notice the skin is red and raw. It's not pleasant to look at, and definitely not pleasant to feel. Some blood might even show. You have a classic case of **chafing**.

LOCKER ROOM LINGO

We simply call it **"the pits"** or **"sandpaper thighs."**

THE RISK RATING

There's lots of discomfort involved with this injury, but no permanent danger.

THE GAME

A likely scenario: It's a hot, humid day but you cannot resist the call of the open road. Primarily, you don't think it's wise to alter your daily pattern of exercise, which includes a long, moderately paced run. But immediately your shirt becomes wet, clingy, and uncomfortable. As you run, you tug at it to allow some air flow across your skin, but the pumping action of your arms quickly returns the shirt to its annoying posi-

159

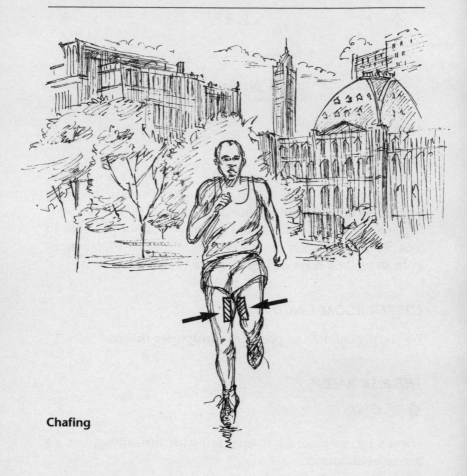

Chafing

tion. After a while, it feels as if someone has put a piece of sandpaper under your arm. For a while, for relief, you run with your arm raised over your head. But that becomes not only very uncomfortable but embarrassing to you as several motorists brake their cars, thinking you are hailing them in need of assistance. It's time for you to retreat home—walking—to make a pit stop. It might appear to be a wimp-out situation. But take heart—it even happens to the best of marathoners on occasion.

THE FIRST DAY TREATMENT

IMPORTANT: **Take a Pit Stop for a Lube Job**

If you have access to petroleum jelly or another lubricating gel, glob it on the affected area. It will minimize the friction and likely you'll be able to resume your sporting activity immediately.

IMPORTANT: **Change of Clothing**

If the chafing is caused by the clothing you're wearing, try a different fit or a different fabric.

RETURN TO ACTION

As soon as you feel comfortable.

REHAB AND PREVENTION

If it's a repetitive problem, you might want to always lube up before you exercise. Coat the area with petroleum jelly or another lubricating gel.

If you're hairy, shave the affected area. Keeping it smooth will lessen the friction.

Be certain your clothing fits properly. That could be a trial-and-error process. Sometimes if the clothing is too tight, it causes chafing. Sometimes clothing that is too loose and bunches up creates the same kind of adverse and painful result.

The problem is less likely to occur in cooler weather. Heat and humidity cause skin to be softer, and therefore more susceptible to irritation from repetitive rubbing.

REHAB AND PREVENTION REVIEW

◆ Lube up!
◆ Have a close shave!
◆ A change of clothes!

Calluses

THE PAIN

There is a slight discomfort under the heel or ball of your foot. You sense there is a swelling there, or that the skin has thickened. The area affected might be as small as a dime, or possibly covers most of your foot. To the touch, you can feel the hardened skin. The more you are on your feet moving about, the more painful it becomes. You have to be active, but not necessarily hyperactive, to suffer from this problem whose medical name is **hyperkeratosis**.

LOCKER ROOM LINGO

When you use the term **callus** you are not being callous or indifferent! It's the only description to use. If your friends react in a callous way, a slight kick with your troubled foot is a permissible response according to our interpretive reading of the Marquis of Queensberry rules.

Note: Because there are so many similarities between a callus and a corn, refer to the Corns section for more details.

THE INSIDE STORY

This inside story is really a skinside story. Reacting to excessive rubbing or pressure, the body has generated more skin cells. This thickening mass of dead skin is, at first, a protective mechanism, but soon becomes a thorny problem.

THE RISK RATING

There's no danger of long-term harm.

THE GAME

A likely scenario: A friend who seeks to explore a wide range
of exercise options convinces you to take Jazzercise. Reluctant at first, you find the rhythms contagious and the movements aerobically challenging. Your friends, who tend
toward more traditional exercise routines, are disdainful and
dismissive of your new routine. But you press on, delighted
with your newly acquired skills, increased energy, and more
sculptured physique. During one hot number requiring some
fancy and rapid footwork, something doesn't feel quite right
on the bottom of your foot. The beat goes on and the symp-

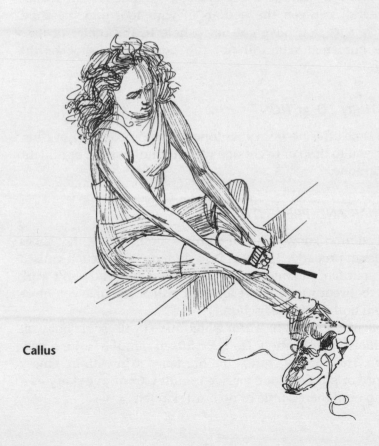

Callus

toms get worse. It's not enough of a problem to force you to sit this one out, but when the number ends you anxiously remove one of your shoes. As your finger traces the hardened skin on your foot, you can't help but wonder whether some of history's most famous dancing feet—Fred Astaire's or Ginger Rogers's—ever suffered the ignominy resulting from callused feet.

THE FIRST DAY TREATMENT

IMPORTANT: **Take the Pressure Off**

Make a "donut" by inserting a small piece of feltlike material between the bottom of your foot and the shoe. Make sure you have cut out a hole in the center of it so the hardened skin will not rub against the shoe or the donut.

RETURN TO ACTION

No time off is necessary, as long as the problem is not causing you to limp or to change your normal posture or athletic technique.

REHAB AND PREVENTION

Any dancer knows, and any athlete should know, that shoes must fit properly. The goal is to decrease the friction caused by your foot rubbing against your shoe. If that doesn't work try footwear with a wider toe area, which will give you more room and minimize friction.

Soak your foot in warm water mixed with some baby oil or moisturizing lotion. Do it for fifteen minutes around bedtime. Then gently "sand" the hardened skin with an emery board or pumice stone for five minutes. Continue every evening until there's little or no hard skin left.

As long as the symptom persists use the donut as recommended in the Treatment section. Use a firmer inner sole, which will help eliminate friction between your foot and shoe.

If it's a recurring problem sprinkle some powder in your shoe, or coat your foot with a skin softener or lubricant whenever you participate in an athletic activity.

Wearing two pairs of socks, one thinner than the other, may help solve the problem. The thinner pair should be worn closest to your foot.

REHAB AND PREVENTION REVIEW

◆ If the shoe fits!
◆ Sand it!
◆ Cushion it!
◆ Grease it!
◆ Take a powder!
◆ Use a donut!
◆ Sock it!

Corns

THE PAIN

The troubled area is on the bottom of your foot, on the top of one or more toes, or between the toes. It hurt a little at first, but the pain intensified. It was clear to you that "something" was there. A pebble? A thorn? When you probed the area with your fingers, you felt an extremely hard, center core. No, it's not a callus. The hard core means you've got a **corn**. Calluses and corns are part of a problem the medical books call **hyperkeratosis**.

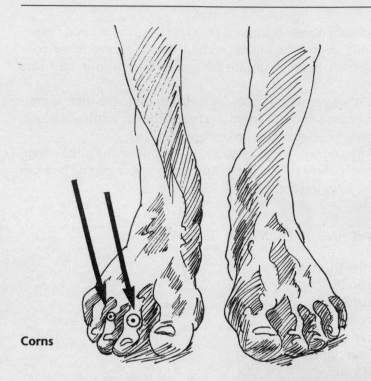

Corns

LOCKER ROOM LINGO

A **corn** sounds a bit dainty, as if it were coming from a seventeenth-century Frenchwoman whose high heels were too tight when she danced the minuet. You can respond by being as corny as you want. But there's no better way of describing the problem.

Note: Because there are so many similarities between a callus and a corn, refer to the Calluses section for more details. However, to the First Day Treatment section, add the following:

IMPORTANT: **Be a Softy**

If the problem is between your toes, separate them with a tuft of cotton.

AN IMPORTANT IDEA: Cushion It

Handle a callus or corn on the top of your toes by padding them with a soft, flat piece of gauze.

And add to the Rehab and Prevention section:

If you are getting corns on the top of your toes or in between them, stretch out your shoe with a shoe tree.

Blisters

THE PAIN

You probably first felt an annoying rubbing sensation between your foot and your shoes, or between your hand and a racquet, oar, or bat. Soon it probably became more painful, as if someone had touched the area with a lighted cigarette or had rubbed salt on raw skin. It's a familiar problem to anyone who has spent a significant amount of time trying to recapture the Glory Days. And when you look at it, there's no doubt you have a **blister**. Sometimes blisters are huge. You might think yours deserves its own zip code.

LOCKER ROOM LINGO

"**Blister**" is the unalterable name. There's no locker room substitute. It's an ironic name because, as you have learned, there's certainly no bliss to be found in having a blister.

THE INSIDE STORY

Friction is the culprit. The body has responded by creating a sac of serous fluid. The bulging sac is painful because of the pressure it puts on the inner layers of the skin.

THE RISK RATING

There is a risk of infection if not handled properly.

THE GAME

A likely scenario: Your shiny, new Rollerblades have doubled the distance you usually cover along the curving, cement pathways of your favorite woodland retreat. About twenty minutes into the ride, your attention is repeatedly drawn away from the flora and fauna to your foot. You wiggle it, but it's impossible to ease the friction that seems to be developing along the outer edge of your big toe. The rigid construction of the shoe is no help in making your foot feel comfortable. Another half mile on the path and there's no doubt that a blister has formed on your toe and is getting larger and more painful the more you skate. When you double back to your

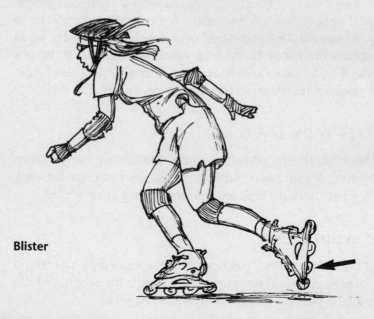

Blister

starting point, the discomfort is almost disabling, and intensifies as you remove the skate, which momentarily puts even more pressure on the troubled area. You react by using some blistering language.

THE FIRST DAY TREATMENT

IMMEDIATE: **Take the Pressure Off**

If the blister is still whole, it's best to leave it alone if possible. Certainly do not break it by pinching, popping, or piercing it with an unsterile pointed object. That could cause an infection. It's best to let the blister heal on its own. Relieve the pain by surrounding the blister with a donut. No, not the edible kind, but a small bit of padding to keep the affected area separated from whatever it was rubbing against. Commercially available donuts are perfect for the job.

If an unbroken blister proves to be disabling, draining it is permissible. Pierce it with a sterile needle. Allow all of the fluid to drain. **Do not remove the skin.** The skin will act as a "biological bandage." Put some antibiotic ointment on the area and then cover it with a store-bought sterile pad.

If the blister burst during your athletic activity, immediately clean and dry the area. An over-the-counter antibiotic ointment will help prevent infection. Cover the open wound with an adhesive bandage.

▶ CAUTION: It's important to monitor the blister area for any redness that would indicate an infection. An unattended blister can lead to a big enough problem that could ground you for longer than you'd like.

RETURN TO ACTION

If you can tolerate the discomfort, then play through the pain. But any sign of infection is a stop sign, too. Most blisters will clear up within a few days.

REHAB AND PREVENTION

Continue to use the donut technique until all the discomfort has passed.

You can reduce the friction that causes blisters on your feet by wearing two pairs of socks. The sock closest to your skin should be as thin as possible. Good old petroleum jelly, rubbed on the most susceptible areas of your feet, may also do the trick.

If your feet have a tendency to perspire excessively, use an absorbent powder.

Athletic footwear that is too big, too small, or too worn out is not foot friendly. Do your feet a favor. Always wear footwear that fits properly! Be certain the tongue of your shoe is straight and wrinkle free. Adjust your laces. Being footloose won't necessarily mean you'll be blister free. The reverse is also true. Laces that are too tight can also cause blisters.

If the blister is on your hand, use talcum powder before you pick up your bat or racquet. Or wear a glove especially designed for your kind of sport.

REHAB AND PREVENTION REVIEW

◆ Keep the pressure off!
◆ Reduce the friction!
◆ Dry out!
◆ If the shoe doesn't fit, don't wear it!

Jogger's Nipples

THE PAIN

As you exercised, you felt a raw, burning sensation in your nipples. At your first opportunity, you might have stopped and lifted your shirt to check out the problem. If you decided to put your shirt back on and complete your activity, you might soon have found the condition had worsened and that your nipples had begun to bleed. Your sweat makes the problem even more painful. And if you tried to cool off in a shower, the beads of water hitting your chest no doubt felt like needles piercing the skin around your nipples. It may be surprising to you, but male jocks are more susceptible to the problem than female jocks, because bras minimize the friction that causes **"mechanical irritation of the nipples."**

LOCKER ROOM LINGO

If you tell your Glory Days colleagues that you're suffering from **"jogger's nipples"** they might respond with some racy locker room humor. But don't retreat. You're using the generally accepted term for the problem.

THE RISK RATING

It's annoying, maybe even embarrassing, but not a long-term threat.

THE GAME

A likely scenario: This is going to be your day for distance. You have carved out enough time for a long, leisurely run that you expect will help you prepare—physically and mentally—for the marathon you have long dreamed of entering. The weather is warm and humid, and a film of sweat quickly flushes over your entire body. Your running top darkens with moisture and begins to cling to you. With each swing of your arms, you feel an annoying irritation—a burning sensation—in your nipples. You tug at your shirt to stretch it away from your chest, but the relief is only momentary. You tough

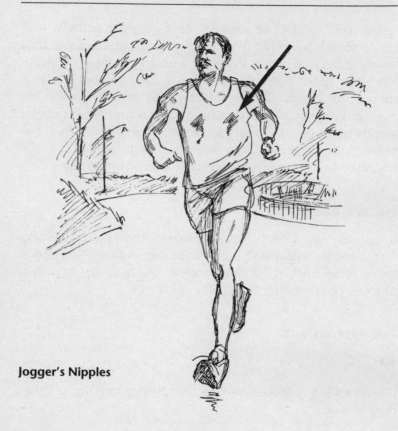

Jogger's Nipples

it out, but soon there is a show of red on your shirt. Your chafed nipples have begun to bleed. No doubt about it—you have **jogger's nipples.**

THE FIRST DAY TREATMENT

IMMEDIATE: Grin and Bear It

Although the sight of blood on your shirt can be frightening, this is a simple problem to resolve. If you can't run shirtless the quick resolution to the problem is to cut this run short. It's the constant rubbing of your shirt that has created the problem. If you can run bare-chested, do so.

RETURN TO ACTION

As soon as you're able to do so comfortably.

REHAB AND PREVENTION

Get the shirt off your back! A different style, a different size, or a different material might do the trick. You might try wearing a shirt that does not have a decal or lettering on the front. Sometimes that stiffens the shirt and increases the likelihood of irritation.

Lubing up—smearing petroleum jelly or another lubricant on your nipples before you run—will decrease chafing.

Putting a gauze pad over each nipple will also help. But be careful how you tape it on. If you have a hairy chest, the removal process might be a sticky and painful problem.

REHAB AND PREVENTION REVIEW

◆ Style check!
◆ Lube up!
◆ Cover up!

Heat Exhaustion

THE PAIN

On a blast furnace kind of summer's day, gulping for air, you wobbled and weaved toward the shade of a tree. Hot, dizzy, faint, crampy, nauseous, thirsty, and shedding moisture like a wet sponge tightly squeezed, you hardly exemplify your self-image of an uncompromising all-weather athlete. Yes, the mind was willing, but your body has succumbed to **heat exhaustion.**

LOCKER ROOM LINGO

The term heat exhaustion hardly seems to have a place in a locker room vocabulary. It might sound so pedestrian, one manifestation of being elderly, overweight, and out of shape. Not so! We heard one youthful, trim victim, in search of verbal satisfaction, refer to it as a **"flame out."** Sounds good to us.

THE INSIDE STORY

When you sweat, the moisture that flows onto your skin evaporates, taking heat away from your body. If you don't drink up to replace what you're losing, you will begin to sweat less. That will make it difficult for your body to cool off. That's when your troubles begin. Also, in the sweat that pours out of you are essential water and body salts that include sodium, potassium, and chloride, which are essential to the proper functioning of muscles and nerves.

THE RISK RATING

This injury should not be ignored. It can lead to heat stroke, which can be deadly.

THE GAME

A likely scenario: You pride yourself as being undeterred by the elements. In fact, you find adverse conditions enticing. Running when no one else is out there brings you great satisfaction. A mental enhancement of your physical achievement. You have long thought the therapeutic benefits of exercise are as much mental as physical. Few psychologists would disagree. But, there's a limit! And this time you have exceeded it.

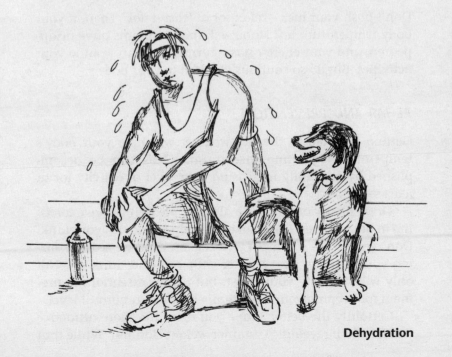

Dehydration

THE FIRST DAY TREATMENT

IMMEDIATE: **Halt**

This is not optional! At the first signs of excessive thirst and sweating, dizziness, nausea, and feeling faint, stop to cool off.

IMMEDIATE: **Shade**

Get out of the sun and find a cool spot to get your temperature down.

IMMEDIATE: **Drink Up**

It's important to *immediately* replenish the fluids lost by sweating. It's important that the fluids should contain sodium, potassium, and chloride.

RETURN TO ACTION

Don't push your luck—relax for at least a day. Then, if your body temperature has stabilized, the symptoms have disappeared, and your energy has returned you can resume your activities. But do so cautiously! Listen to your body.

REHAB AND PREVENTION

Getting adjusted to the hot weather will help your body's temperature-regulating mechanisms. This can be accomplished by gradually increasing your level of activity for at least seven days.

Drink plenty of fluids (no alcohol, please!) before exercising in hot weather. Don't take just a sip or two. Fill your tank. Don't feel you're a wimp if you take time out for a drink during your activity. Carry water with you and drink up. Not only will it satisfy your thirst, but it's an essential requirement for keeping your body temperature at a normal level.

Certainly the better shape you're in, the more attractive you'll look in revealing, summer-weight clothing. While that may be of paramount importance to you, remember also that the better your conditioning, the more able you are to withstand the debilitating effects of hot weather.

REHAB AND PREVENTION REVIEW

◆ Get used to the heat!
◆ Get in better shape!
◆ Get more fluids into your system!
◆ Take frequent breaks!

Muscle Cramps

THE PAIN

You could feel it begin to happen but didn't know how to stop it. A sudden tightening. A knot forming. The pain quickly reaching a crescendo and then easing off. A soreness remains. When you rub it firmly, the pain increases for the moment. You're suffering from a cramp, which can occur in any muscle of your body.

LOCKER ROOM LINGO

We don't know who Charley was, or how his horse got into the act, but **charley horse** is the all-purpose name for a cramp.

THE INSIDE STORY

Salts and other electrolytes (sodium, potassium, and chloride) are important for the contraction and movement of muscle fibers. These electrolytes act like electrical charges enabling your muscles to contract and relax. During long periods of exercise, especially in hot conditions, excessive sweating depletes your body fluids, including precious electrolytes. This creates an electrolyte imbalance in the fluids in and around your muscle and nerve fibers, causing spontaneous contractions and a subsequent inability to then relax the tightened muscle.

THE RISK RATING

Usually a cramp is nothing to worry about and will disappear with a minimum of care.

▶ CAUTION: If a cramp occurs during high heat, while you're sweating excessively, accompanied by dizziness or extreme thirst, it could be a warning sign that you are suffering from dehydration.

THE GAME

You're in the pool for your daily exercise, aggressively using your legs, flutter kicking to keep up with the swimmer in the

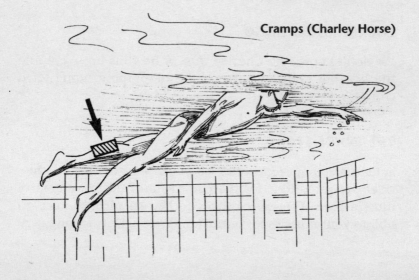

Cramps (Charley Horse)

next lane. You've been taught that the proper kick is performed by keeping your knees straight and your toes pointed. Seeing the competition with an increasing lead, you work harder, tightening your calf to generate a more powerful kick. That's when you suddenly feel your calf muscle tightening into a ball. The pain is excruciating, and the race is over.

THE FIRST DAY TREATMENT

IMMEDIATE: **Slow It Down**

Your cramps may be the result of overexertion, so take it easy. This just may be enough to resolve the problem.

IMMEDIATE: **Stretch It Out**

Slowly stretching the cramped muscles can be very effective. Example: If you have a charley horse in your leg, stretch your foot, moving your toes back in the direction of the pain. Hold the stretch until the cramp eases.

IMMEDIATE: **Massage It**

Massage the cramp by pressing your fingers into the affected muscle, gently kneading it.

RETURN TO ACTION

If you can tolerate the pain there's no problem trying to continue with your physical activity. If you do stop, feel free to return anytime.

REHAB AND PREVENTION

Warm up by slowly getting into your activity. If you're a swimmer, take a few easy laps. If you're a runner, take a light jog for a few minutes. If you're a cyclist, take an easy ride for ten minutes.

Be certain your tank is full. If you tend to sweat a lot, be certain you are not thirsty *before* you begin your sports activity. And take frequent breaks to replenish the fluids you lose *during* the activity.

Know your limits. Trying to push yourself beyond your comfort zone is an invitation to a cramp. Being in proper shape to match the demands of your level of exercise will also minimize overexertion and the chances of cramping.

▶ CAUTION: If you frequently experience muscle cramps while sleeping or just walking you should see a doctor. It may be a sign of a circulation problem.

REHAB AND PREVENTION REVIEW

◆ Warm up!
◆ Drink up!
◆ Know your limits!
◆ Shape up!

Side Stitch

THE PAIN

The pain, just below your rib cage on your right side, is probably something that has occurred on occasion during your athletic career. The discomfort, which could have been acute, probably eased soon after you halted your sports activity. Unless you somehow misplaced a knitting needle that was jabbing you as you ran, you have a **side stitch.** A side stitch can also occur on your left side, or even be felt in your shoulder, but those are less common. Running is its most common ignition factor, but it has been known to occur in other sports where the body is jarred up and down, including motor biking.

LOCKER ROOM LINGO

The references to this kind of pain are quite limited to nothing more anatomical or poetic than a **"side stitch"** or just a **"stitch."** Simple but profound, everyone will know what you're talking about.

THE INSIDE STORY

Why your body "stitches" is a mystery. While there are several theories, its cause is not fully understood. It's generally thought to be a spasm of your diaphragm caused by an irregular breathing pattern, poor conditioning, or possibly eating too close to the time you begin your physical activity.

THE RISK RATING

It will eventually go away on its own. There's no known risk factor even if you repeatedly try to run through the pain.

THE GAME

A likely scenario: You choose a familiar path and a familiar regimen. There are no surprises as you run effortlessly, keeping track of distance by the recognition of what have, by now, become spiritual landmarks. The mottled elm expressing strength and courageous indifference to time at the half mile. The rugged stone wall berthing territorial integrity at the mile. A half mile further, at the bend, a rutted wagon path marking entry to a lilac-perfumed cemetery. Then, a mile to the village fountain, and its simple granite-edged preachment about generosity to man and mule. But this run of physical and psychological gratification is suddenly interrupted by a pain not felt in many years. Nevertheless, it's so

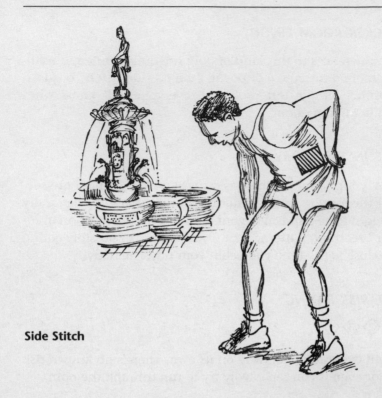

Side Stitch

familiar: the side stitch. It has pierced the mood of the moment without warning. There is no way to ignore it.

THE FIRST DAY TREATMENT

OPTIONAL: **A Change of Pace**

Chances are a few minutes' rest or slowing your pace will ease the discomfort. If you want to gut it out by running through the pain, try taking slower and deeper breaths.

OPTIONAL: **Put On the Pressure**

As you gallop along, gentle pressure applied to the painful area with your fingertips may gradually help.

OPTIONAL: **Get a Leg Up**

If the pain persists even after you halt your activity, lie down on your back and, if you can, lift your feet up and back over your head. This will eliminate the stress on your stomach and internal organs.

RETURN TO ACTION

If you have to stop, try to resume your activity soon after the stitch disappears. If exercise keeps you in stitches, stop for a longer period of time and try again.

Note: Some residual soreness may last for a few days.

REHAB AND PREVENTION

Anyone suffering side stitches might be reminded of the old adage "Never exercise soon after eating." It's wise to wait at least two hours!

Control your running regimen. Run at a comfortable pace. What's comfortable? If you can easily hold a conversation while running, you've achieved the goal.

Proper breathing is a great benefit not only to athletes but to public speakers as well. Good athletes and exceptional speakers practice the same way. Lie down on your back. Place your hands on your stomach, and breathe from the diaphragm. Your chest should not heave, but your hands should be moving up and down as you breathe in and out. Practice until you can breathe this way naturally.

It's important to have strong abdominal muscles. It's a way to possibly help prevent side stitches, and a good way to help thwart back problems.

REHAB AND PREVENTION REVIEW

- ◆ Don't eat and run!
- ◆ Run with your head, not over it!

- ◆ Learn how to breathe!
- ◆ Firm up!

THE EXERCISES

Abdomen strengthen: 1 ◆ 2 ◆ 3 ◆ 4

Part Four

---◆---

STRETCHES
AND
STRENGTHENING
EXERCISES

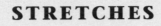

STRETCHES

Neck

STRETCH ◆ 1

NAME: The flexion-extension stretch.

TARGET: Front and back muscles of the neck.

STARTING POSITION: Sit straight up in a chair. Relax your shoulders, and place your hands down by your side.

THE MOTION: Looking straight ahead, bring your chin to your chest.

Hold for a count of one.

Lift your head all the way up, so that you are looking at the ceiling.

Hold for a count of one.

REPETITIONS: Do this exercise twenty times.

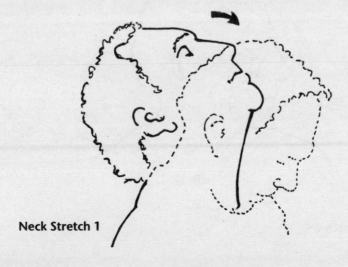

Neck Stretch 1

STRETCH ◆ **2**

NAME: The rotation stretch.

TARGET: Rotator muscles of the neck.

STARTING POSITION: Sit straight up in a chair. Relax your shoulders and place your hands down by your side.

THE MOTION: Look straight ahead, then slowly turn your head to the right.
   Hold for a count of one.
   Slowly turn your head to the left side.
   Hold for a count of one.

REPETITIONS: Do this exercise twenty times.

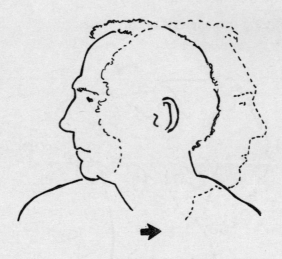

Neck Stretch 2

STRETCH ◆ 3

NAME: The side-to-side stretch.

TARGET: Upper trapezius and levator scapulae muscles. These are the muscles of the lower neck and upper back.

STARTING POSITION: Sit straight up in a chair. Relax your shoulders, keeping your hands down by your side.

THE MOTION: Looking straight ahead, slowly bring your right ear to your shoulder.
   Hold for a count of one.
   Slowly bring your left ear to your shoulder.
   Hold for a count of one.

REPETITIONS: Do each side twenty times.

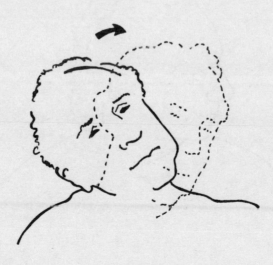

Neck Stretch 3

STRETCH ◆ **4**

NAME: Semicircle stretch.

TARGET: All neck muscles.

STARTING POSITION: Sit straight up in a chair.

THE MOTION: While relaxing your shoulders, keeping your hands down by your side, and looking straight ahead, bring your chin to your chest. Slowly swing your chin to the right.
    Hold for a count of one.
    Swing your chin over to the left side.
    Hold for a count of one.

REPETITIONS: Perform twenty times on each side.

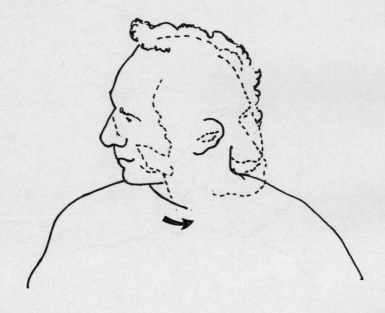

Neck Stretch 4

STRETCH ◆ 5

NAME: Shoulder shrugs.

TARGET: Upper trapezius and levator scapulae muscles. These are the muscles of the lower neck and upper back.

STARTING POSITION: Sit straight up in a chair. Relax your shoulders, keeping your hands down by your side.

THE MOTION: Slowly shrug both shoulders upwards.
    Hold for a count of five.
    Slowly lower your shoulders to their relaxed level.

REPETITIONS: Perform ten times.

STRETCH ◆ 6

NAME: Shoulder circle stretch.

TARGET: Most neck and shoulder muscles.

STARTING POSITION: Sit straight up in a chair. Relax your shoulders and keep your hands down by your side.

THE MOTION: In a circular motion:
    Slowly shrug both shoulders upward.
    Move shoulders forward.
    Move shoulders backward.

REPETITIONS: Perform the exercise ten times. Reverse direction, and do ten more.

Shoulder

STRETCH ◆ 1

NAME: Towel stretch.

TARGET: Rotator cuff muscles. These deep shoulder muscles are used whenever you move your arm.

STARTING POSITION: Stand up straight. Drape a bath towel over your good side shoulder.

THE MOTION: Grasp the front end of the towel with your good side hand. Grasp the other end, which is behind you, with your trouble side hand. With your good side hand, pull the

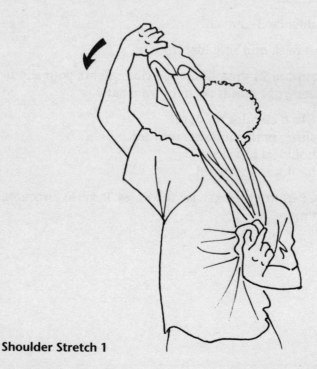

Shoulder Stretch 1

towel down toward your waist. Allow the arm behind you to be pulled up toward your neck. Hold for five seconds.

REPETITIONS: Perform ten of these exercises. Relax for ten seconds between repetitions.

Remember to keep your back straight. If you feel increased pain in your shoulder, lower your trouble side arm by loosening the towel.

STRETCH ◆ 2

NAME: Outward rotation stretch.

TARGET: Rotator cuff muscles.

STARTING POSITION: Lie down on your back. Your trouble side arm should be extended up and out from your side at shoulder height.

THE MOTION: Bend that elbow ninety degrees back toward your body. Keep your elbow on the floor, and move your forearm (the area from the elbow to the hand) backwards as far as you can. It might help if you have some weight (a soup can will do nicely) in that hand. Hold for five seconds.

REPETITIONS: Perform ten of these exercises. Rest ten seconds between each exercise.

Keep your shoulder flat on the surface. Stop immediately if you feel any pain.

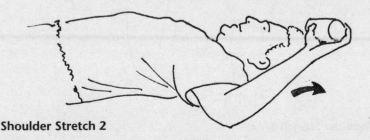

Shoulder Stretch 2

STRETCH ◆ 3

NAME: Stick stretch.

TARGET: Pectoral muscles. These chest muscles are used when you lift your arms.

STARTING POSITION: Stand up straight. Rest a broomstick, a baseball bat, or a similar length of wood on the back of your shoulders.

THE MOTION: Put your arms behind the stick and drape them over the top.

Slowly slide the stick down your back until you feel tension in your chest.

Hold for a count of thirty seconds, then roll it back up to its starting position.

REPETITIONS: Do it five times, resting for a count of twenty between each one.

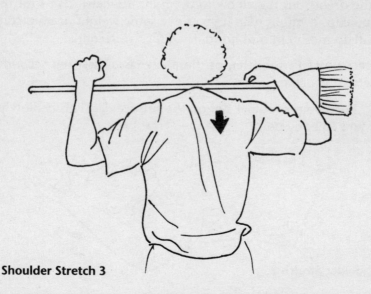

Shoulder Stretch 3

STRETCH ◆ **4**

NAME: Over-the-head stretch.

TARGET: Latissimus dorsi and lower trapezius muscles. These muscles are mainly used to support your back when you're lifting something.

STARTING POSITION: Raise the arm to be stretched over your head.

THE MOTION: Grab that elbow with your other hand and pull the elbow closer to your head. Hold for a count of fifteen.

REPETITIONS: Do this exercise five times, resting for a count of twenty in between.

Stop if this exercise produces pain in your shoulder.

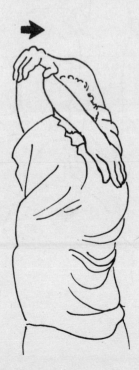

Shoulder Stretch 4

STRETCH ◆ 5

NAME: Arm crossover stretch.

TARGET: Middle trapezius muscles. These are part of the support system of your back.

STARTING POSITION: Stand up and cross the arm to be stretched across your chest.

THE MOTION: Grab that elbow with your other hand.

Pull the stretching arm as far as you can across your chest and hold for a count of twenty.

REPETITIONS: Do it five times, resting for a count of ten seconds between repetitions.

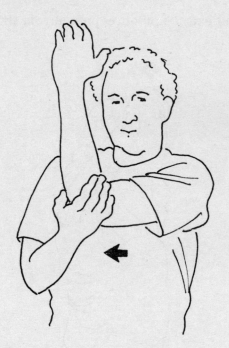

Shoulder Stretch 5

STRETCH ◆ **6**

NAME: Pulley stretch.

TARGET: Shoulder joint.

For this stretch you'll have to make a trip to a sporting goods store. Ask for a set of overhead pulleys, which can be attached over a door.

STARTING POSITION: Sit on a chair.

THE MOTION: Grab the pulley handles and gently pull down with the hand of your uninjured side.

Allow your other arm to be pulled up over your head as far as you can tolerate. It will be painful but that's okay.

Hold for a count of three, then reverse direction to starting position.

REPETITIONS: Do fifty times.

STRETCH ◆ **7**

NAME: Forward arm-lift stretch.

TARGET: Shoulder joint.

STARTING POSITION: Lie down on your back and fold your hands on your stomach.

THE MOTION: Use your good side hand to slowly help lift the bad side hand to the point of pain, or over your head if you can.

Hold for five seconds, then slowly return to the starting position.

REPETITIONS: Perform ten times, resting for a count of ten seconds between repetitions.

This is one of the few exercises where it's beneficial to experience some pain.

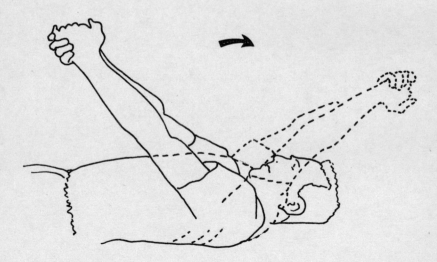

Shoulder Stretch 7

STRETCH ◆ 8

NAME: Pendulum stretch.

TARGET: Shoulder joint.

STARTING POSITION: Stand up straight. Hold a weight, up to five pounds (a soup can is fine), in the hand of your injured side.

THE MOTION: Bend from the waist so that your arm hangs down in front of you.
   Gently swing your arm forward and backward.
   Then gently swing it from side to side.

REPETITIONS: Do the forward and backward motion fifty times. Rest for a few moments, then perform the side-to-side motion fifty times.

You may want to support yourself by placing your good hand on a table. Stop if you experience any pain in your shoulder.

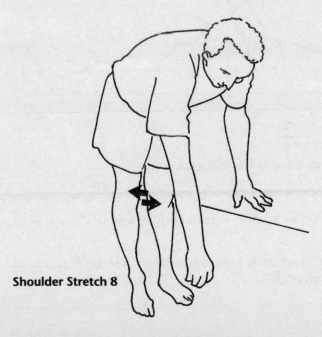

Shoulder Stretch 8

Back

STRETCH ◆ 1

NAME: Single knee to chest stretch.

TARGET: Low back muscles.

STARTING POSITION: Choose a firm surface and lie flat on your back.

THE MOTION: Bring one knee up as far as you can toward your chest. The other leg should stay extended flat on the surface.
  Hold this position for a count of thirty.
  Switch legs and repeat exercise.

REPETITIONS: Do five times with each leg.

Back Stretch 1

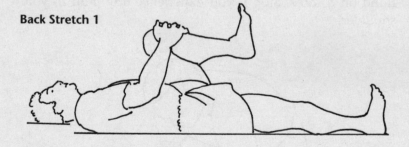

STRETCH ◆ 2

NAME: Double knee to chest stretch.

TARGET: Low back muscles.

STARTING POSITION: Choose a firm surface and lie flat on your back.

THE MOTION: Bend both knees, bringing them back as far as you can to your chest.

Cradle knees with your arms and hold for a count of thirty.

REPETITIONS: Do five times.

Back Stretch 2

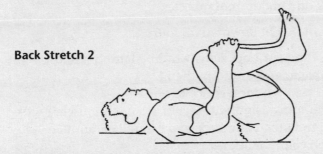

STRETCH ◆ **3**

NAME: Trunk roll stretch.

TARGET: Rotator muscles of lower back.

STARTING POSITION: Choose firm surface and lie flat on your back.

THE MOTION: Bend both knees up far enough so that your feet are flat on the floor.

Move both knees over to one side as far as you can and hold for a count of three.

Reverse directions and repeat the exercise.

REPETITIONS: Do five times in each direction.

Back Stretch 3

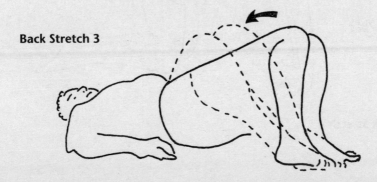

STRETCH ◆ **4**

NAME: Cat and camel stretch.

TARGET: Back and abdominal muscles.

STARTING POSITION: Get down on all fours.

THE MOTION: Dip your back downward by letting it relax. You should be able to look straight ahead.

Hold this position for a count of one.

Now simultaneously tighten your stomach muscles, look downward, and arch your back in a humplike manner.

Hold for a count of one.

REPETITIONS: Do fifteen times.

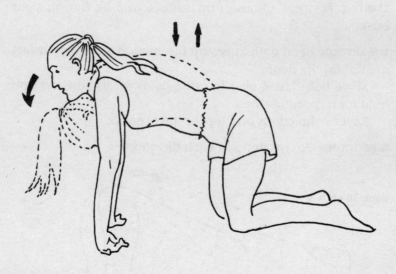

Back Stretch 4

Wrist

STRETCH ◆ 1

NAME: Downward wrist stretch.

TARGET: Extensor muscles of wrist and hand. These muscles help you to lift your wrist and hand and to bend your elbow.

STARTING POSITION: Sit or stand with your trouble side arm fully extended in front of you, palm down.

THE MOTION: Push your trouble side hand down from the wrist only by applying pressure with your good hand.
Hold for ten seconds.

REPETITIONS: Perform ten times, resting for ten seconds between exercises.

Do not bend wrist to the point of pain. If you feel any pain while doing this exercise, stop immediately.

Wrist Stretch 1

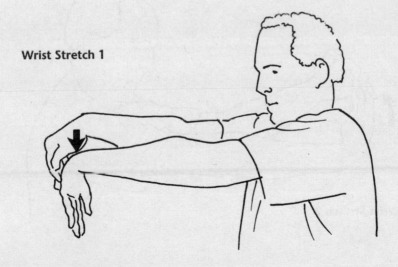

STRETCH ◆ 2

NAME: Upward wrist stretch.

TARGET: Flexor muscles of wrist and hand. These muscles help to bend your wrist, hand, and elbow.

STARTING POSITION: Sit or stand with your trouble side arm fully extended in front of you, palm down.

THE MOTION: With your good hand, push the other hand at the wrist up and backwards.

Hold for a count of ten.

REPETITIONS: Do the stretch ten times.

Do not go past the point that causes you pain—if this exercise can't be accomplished without feeling pain, stop immediately.

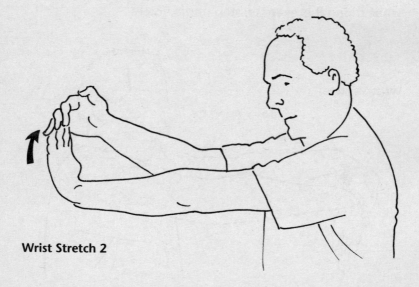

Wrist Stretch 2

Finger

STRETCH ◆ 1

NAME: Hand ballet.

TARGET: Intrinsic muscles of the hand and fingers. These muscles, located in the hand, are responsible for hand and finger movements.

STARTING POSITION: Point your hand and fingers upward as if you're about to give a high five.

THE MOTION: Bend your fingers at the first knuckle so they are at a right angle with your palm. Hold for a count of one.
   Curl fingers into a fist. Hold for a count of one.
   Slide fingers up your palm as far as you can. Hold for a count of one.
   Straighten fingers.

REPETITIONS: Do entire exercise five times.

Hip and Thigh

STRETCH ◆ 1

NAME: Back of thigh stretch.

TARGET: Hamstrings. These muscles help your thigh move backward and also bend your knee.

STARTING POSITION: Sit up on a hard surface (such as a table, bench, or countertop). Dangle your good leg off to the side and stretch the injured leg out in front of you. Although it may be difficult at first, try to keep that knee straight.

THE MOTION: Drape a towel around the sole of your foot and lean forward.

Keep your back straight and don't hunch your shoulders!!!

While in this position use the towel to pull the top part of your foot back toward your body.

REPETITIONS: Repeat the exercise five times. Hold each stretch for thirty seconds, and rest for ten seconds between each stretch.

Make certain your motions are smooth and fluid. No bouncing or jerky movements. If necessary you can use the floor as your hard surface. If you do, then follow the above instructions for the injured leg. However, relax your good leg while it's flat on the floor but with your knee bent out to the side, away from your body, as if you're making a figure four.

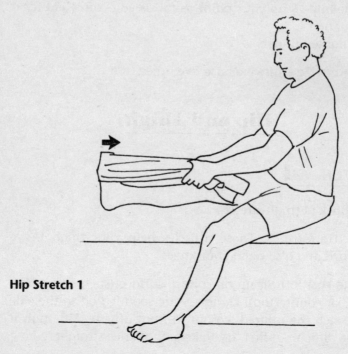

Hip Stretch 1

STRETCH ◆ 2

NAME: Front thigh stretch.

TARGET: Quadriceps. These muscles are used to straighten your leg.

STARTING POSITION: Stand on the leg that does not need to be stretched. Use the opposite hand to balance yourself by holding on to the back of a chair, or by placing your hand against the wall in front of you.

THE MOTION: With your other hand, reach back and grab your trouble side ankle.

Pull your ankle up and backward so that you are also pulling your thigh backward.

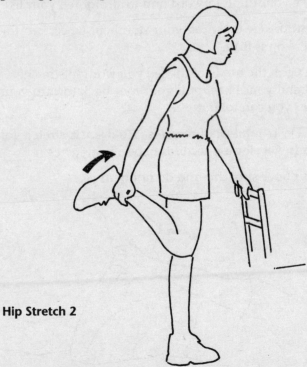

Hip Stretch 2

Keep your back straight and your stomach tight.

If it's easier for you, rest the instep of your foot on a railing behind you. Then lean forward slowly so that you are stretching your thigh.

REPETITIONS: Repeat the exercise five times. Hold each stretch for thirty seconds then rest ten seconds.

Remember to keep your back straight. Do not bounce.

STRETCH ◆ 3

NAME: Rectus femoris stretch.

TARGET: Rectus femoris muscle of the thigh. This muscle is used to move your thigh forward and to straighten your leg.

STARTING POSITION: Lie down on your stomach. Be certain the surface you're on is firm.

THE MOTION: Grab the ankle of the leg you want to stretch.
As you bend your knee, pull your foot back toward your butt as far as you can tolerate.

REPETITIONS: Do a total of three sets. Hold each stretch for thirty seconds. Rest for ten seconds between stretches.

Keep your back straight, and do not bounce.

Hip Stretch 3

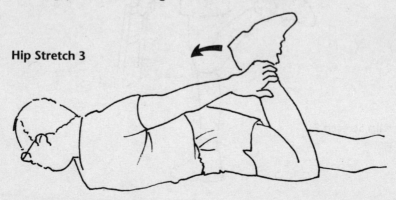

STRETCH ◆ **4**

NAME: Outer thigh stretch.

TARGET: Iliotibial band. This tissue, which travels the outside of your leg from the hip to the knee, aids in bending your leg.

STARTING POSITION: This stretch is different from most you've seen, but it is easy to perform. Sit up, preferably with your back supported against a wall. The leg not being stretched should be straight out in front of you.

THE MOTION: Cross your trouble side leg over your good straight leg, bending that knee so that the heel slides up along the outside of the straight leg.

Grab that knee with the opposite hand and pull it up and across your body.

Hip Stretch 4

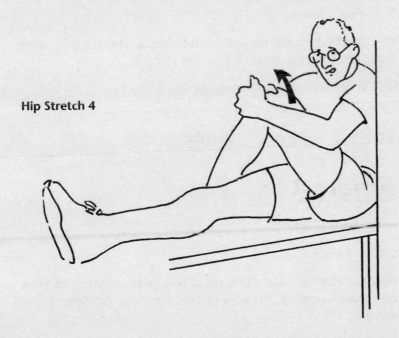

Hold for thirty seconds.
Release and rest ten seconds.

REPETITIONS: Perform the stretch five times.

It's very important to always keep your back straight.

STRETCH ◆ 5

NAME: Groin stretch.

TARGET: Adductor muscles. These inner thigh muscles help you squeeze your legs together.

STARTING POSITION: Sit up and bring the soles of your feet together.

THE MOTION: Lean forward from the hips and grab both your ankles. Keeping your back straight, push down on your knees with your elbows.

REPETITIONS: Perform the stretch five times. Hold it each time for thirty seconds, then rest for ten seconds.

Do not bounce while stretching.

Knee

STRETCH ◆ 1

NAME: Wall slides.

TARGET: Knee joint.

STARTING POSITION: Lie down on a bed or the floor with your butt close to a wall. Put your feet on the wall with your knees straight.

THE MOTION: Slowly lower your injured leg's heel down the wall so that your injured knee bends.

Once you have brought your heel down as far as you can tolerate, hold that position for a count of three.

Slowly lift your injured heel with your good foot until your knee is straight once again.

REPETITIONS: Do fifty times.

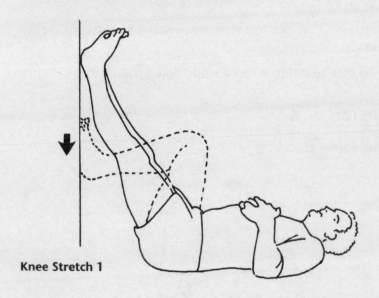

Knee Stretch 1

Leg

STRETCH ◆ 1

NAME: Calf stretch.

TARGET: Gastrocnemius muscles, which help you to move your foot downward. Without them you could not jump. They also help bend your knee.

STARTING POSITION: Stand on a step, curb, or even a pile of books.

THE MOTION: With your hands out in front of you, grab on to a chair or wall for balance.

Let your heels hang down from the edge.

Shift your body weight to your heels—this will force your heels down below the level of your toes.

Hold each stretch for thirty seconds.

REPETITIONS: Perform five stretches, resting in between for ten seconds.

Be careful not to bounce while doing this stretch.

STRETCH ◆ **2**

NAME: Soleus stretch.

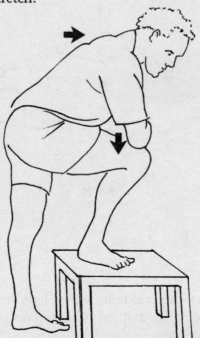

Leg Stretch 2

TARGET: The soleus muscle of the leg, which helps move your foot downward.

STARTING POSITION: You need a chair or table for this stretch.

THE MOTION: Lift your trouble side leg up as if you are about to climb on the chair.
  Be certain your foot is flat on the seat's surface.
  Lean forward so that your body weight is over that foot.

REPETITIONS: Do five stretches, holding each stretch for thirty seconds. Rest ten seconds between stretches.

  Do not bounce or rock your body during this stretch.

STRETCH ◆ **3**

NAME: Front leg stretch.

TARGET: Anterior leg muscles. These muscles lift your foot and toes upward.

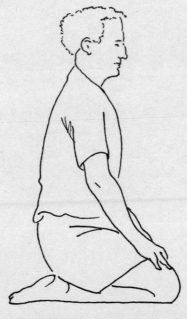

Leg Stretch 3

STARTING POSITION: Kneel on the floor. Point your toes out behind you so that the tops of your feet are in contact with the floor.

THE MOTION: Gently shift your weight backwards as if to sit back onto your heels.

REPETITIONS: Hold each stretch for thirty seconds. Perform the exercise three times, resting ten seconds between each repetition.

If you feel pressure or pain in your knees, kneel on a pillow. Never bounce while doing this exercise.

STRENGTHENING EXERCISES

Shoulder

STRENGTHEN ◆ 1

NAME: Forward arm lift.

TARGET: Anterior deltoid muscle, which is located in your shoulder and helps lift your arm, and the biceps brachii muscles, which help bend your elbow.

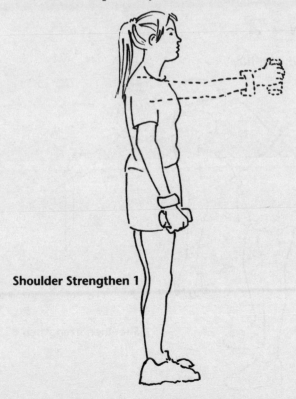

Shoulder Strengthen 1

STARTING POSITION: Stand straight. Put a weight on your trouble side wrist.

THE MOTION: Keep your elbow straight as you lift your arm straight out in front of you.

As you perform this exercise, keep your thumb pointed straight up.

Stop when you reach the level of your shoulder.

Use as much weight as you can handle without causing any pain.

REPETITIONS: Do three sets of ten exercises. Rest for twenty seconds between each set.

Remember—thumbs up!

STRENGTHEN ◆ **2**

NAME: Backward arm lift.

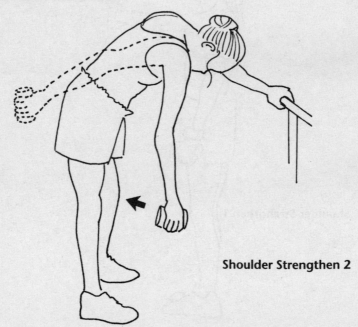

Shoulder Strengthen 2

TARGET: Latissimus dorsi and teres major muscles. These muscles allow your arm to be moved behind you.

STARTING POSITION: Stand erect while doing this exercise.

THE MOTION: Lean forward.

Balance yourself by holding on to a chair or table with the hand you won't be exercising.

Keeping your trouble side arm straight by your side, slowly move your arm back behind you.

Hold for a count of one.

REPETITIONS: Perform three sets of fifteen exercises. Rest twenty seconds between sets.

Use a weight as heavy as you wish as long as it does not cause discomfort in your shoulder or back.

STRENGTHEN ◆ 3

NAME: Arm side lift.

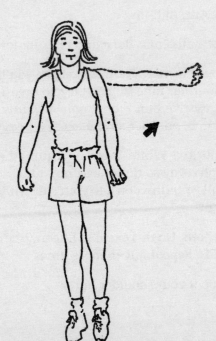

Shoulder Strengthen 3

TARGET: Middle deltoid muscle. This shoulder muscle helps you lift your arm up and out to the side.

STARTING POSITION: Be certain your elbow is straight and your thumb is pointed toward the sky. If you can perform this exercise with a weight on your wrist or in your hand without it causing pain, do so.

THE MOTION: Lift your arm straight out to your side until your arm is level with your shoulder. Work toward a goal of ten pounds.

REPETITIONS: Do the exercise fifteen times. Rest for twenty seconds, then perform fifteen more.

Stop the exercise if your shoulder hurts.

STRENGTHEN ◆ 4

NAME: Arm pull-ins.

TARGET: Latissimus dorsi and teres major muscles.

STARTING POSITION: For this exercise you'll need a rubber cord, an old inner tube from a bicycle tire, a commercially available resistive band, or a pair of panty hose. Attach it to a doorknob, banister, or the leg of a heavy table.

THE MOTION: While standing, grab the cord and step far enough away so that it becomes taut.
Pull your arm down to your side while keeping your elbow straight.

REPETITIONS: Do this exercise fifteen times, then rest for twenty seconds. Repeat fifteen more times.

Stop if your shoulder hurts.

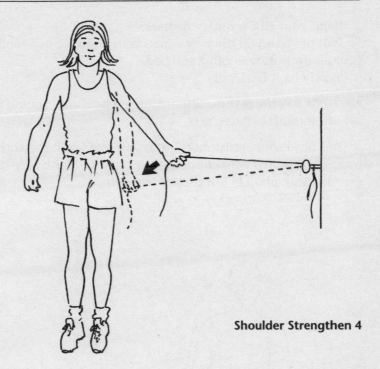

Shoulder Strengthen 4

STRENGTHEN ◆ **5**

NAME: Shoulder inward rotation.

TARGET: Subscapularis muscle of the rotator cuff. This muscle assists in all shoulder movements.

STARTING POSITION: You need an old bicycle inner tube, elastic cord, commercially available resistive band, or a pair of old panty hose for this exercise. Anything elastic that's big enough will work! Attach it to a doorknob, banister, or the leg of a heavy table.

THE MOTION: Stand straight up and hold other end of the elastic in your trouble side hand.

Bend your elbow ninety degrees.
Pull the band all the way across your chest while keeping your elbow tightly against your side.
Slowly let it back out.

REPETITIONS: Perform three sets of fifteen repetitions, resting for twenty seconds between sets.

You need some resistance, but if you can't pull the elastic completely across your chest, the elastic is too tight. Stop this exercise immediately if it causes any pain.

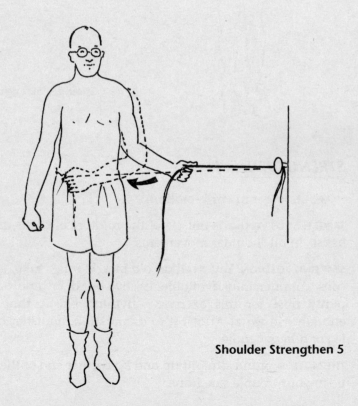

Shoulder Strengthen 5

STRENGTHEN ◆ 6

NAME: Shoulder outward rotation.

TARGET: Supraspinatus, infraspinatus, and teres minor muscles of the rotator cuff. These muscles assist in all shoulder movements.

STARTING POSITION: You will need an old bicycle inner tube, a commercially available resistive band, elastic cord, or a pair of old panty hose for this exercise. Anything elastic that's big enough will do! Attach it to a doorknob, banister, or the leg of a heavy table.

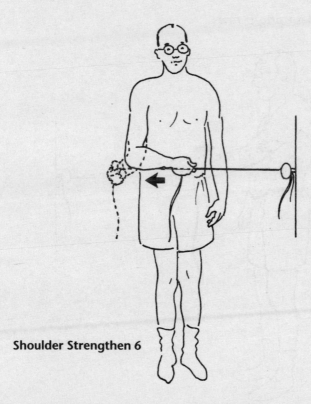

Shoulder Strengthen 6

THE MOTION: Stand straight up with your uninjured side closest to the elastic.

Bend your trouble side elbow ninety degrees.

Grasp the elastic in that hand and pull the elastic away from your body.

Keep that elbow close to your side throughout the motion.

REPETITIONS: Perform three sets of fifteen exercises, resting twenty seconds between sets.

Stop exercise immediately if it produces any pain.

STRENGTHEN ◆ 7

NAME: Shoulder upright rows.

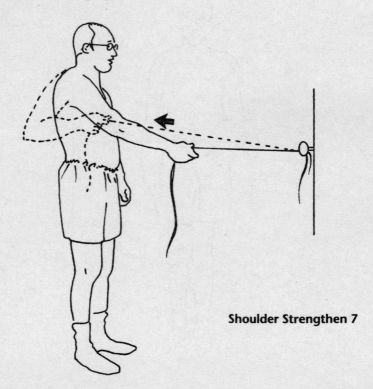

Shoulder Strengthen 7

TARGET: Rhomboid and middle trapezius muscles. These muscles, located in your middle back, provide support for lifting.

STARTING POSITION: You will need an old bicycle inner tube, or a similar commercially available elastic band, attached to a doorknob, banister, or leg of a heavy table.

THE MOTION: Stand with the band in front of you.

Holding the band in your trouble side hand, step back until the band becomes taut.

Raise your arm to shoulder level.

Bending your elbow, pull the band toward you and hold for a count of one.

Then reverse the movement.

Do this fifteen times.

REPETITIONS: Perform three sets of fifteen exercises, resting twenty seconds between sets.

Stop this exercise immediately if you feel any pain.

STRENGTHEN ◆ 8

NAME: Wall push-up.

TARGET: Pectoralis and serratus anterior muscles, which are part of your chest, and the triceps muscles, which are in the back of your arm. These muscles all aid in lifting your arm.

STARTING POSITION: Stand approximately two feet away from a wall. Lean forward and put both hands on the wall in front of you at shoulder level.

THE MOTION: Slowly bend your elbows and lean forward so your chest comes close to the wall.

Hold for a count of one.

Then slowly straighten your arms to push your chest away from the wall.

REPETITIONS: Perform two sets of fifteen. Rest for twenty seconds in between sets.

Back

STRENGTHEN ◆ 1

NAME: Back curl.

TARGET: Erector spinae muscles. These are back muscles used to keep your back straight while sitting and walking.

STARTING POSITION: Lie on your stomach with your arms by your side.

THE MOTION: Slowly lift your head and chest three inches. Hold for a count of one; slowly return to starting position.

REPETITIONS: Do fifteen repetitions, then relax for fifteen seconds. Do two sets.

Stop immediately if you feel any back or neck pain.

Back Strengthen 1

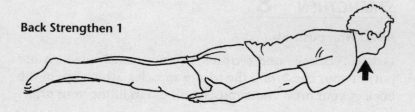

STRENGTHEN ◆ 2

NAME: Prone leg lift.

TARGET: Gluteus maximus, which is the major muscle in your butt, and the hamstrings, which are in the back of your thigh.

STARTING POSITION: Lie on the floor, on your stomach.

THE MOTION: Keeping both legs straight, lift one leg up about six inches.

Do not bend your knee, and do not arch your back.

REPETITIONS: Do a set of fifteen with each leg. Rest for fifteen seconds and do another set.

You can progress with this exercise by adding weights on your ankles. Do not add more than ten pounds on each leg.

Do not lift your leg so high that you begin to arch your back. Stop immediately if you feel back pain.

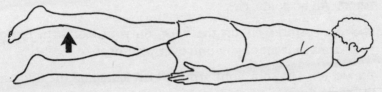

Back Strengthen 2

STRENGTHEN ◆ 3

NAME: Prone arm lift.

TARGET: Trapezius muscles. These are the muscles of your middle and upper back.

STARTING POSITION: Lie on the floor, on your stomach. Bring your arms straight in front of you above your head with your arms pointed upward.

THE MOTION: Lift one arm three inches off of the floor.

Slowly lower to starting position.

Back Strengthen 3

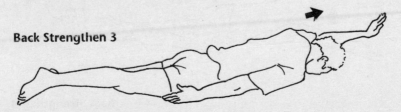

REPETITIONS: Do fifteen with each arm—you can alternate if you like. Rest for fifteen seconds, then do another set of fifteen. You can progress with this exercise by adding weight in your hand. However, do not lift more than five pounds.

Stop if you feel any back pain.

STRENGTHEN ◆ 4

NAME: Prone opposite arm and leg lift.

TARGET: All back muscles.

STARTING POSITION: Lie on the floor, on your stomach. Bring your arms in front of you and over your head.

THE MOTION: Lift your right arm and left leg up off the floor at the same time.
 Hold for a count of one.
 Slowly lower arm and leg back to the starting position.
 Repeat by alternating arm and leg.

REPETITIONS: Do one set of fifteen, then rest for fifteen seconds. Do another set of fifteen. You can progress by adding weight to your arms and legs. No more than five pounds on each arm and ten pounds on each leg should be lifted.

Stop immediately if you feel any pain.

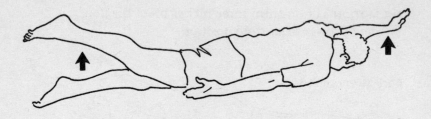

Back Strengthen 4

Abdomen

STRENGTHEN ◆ 1

NAME: 1/2 straight forward sit-up.

TARGET: Rectus abdominus. This muscle located in your abdomen allows you to bend forward from the waist and helps stabilize your back.

STARTING POSITION: Lie on your back on the floor. Bend your knees so your feet are flat on the floor. Cross your arms over your chest (not behind your neck).

THE MOTION: Slowly lift your head and chest halfway between the floor and your knees.

Hold for only one second.

Return to your starting position.

REPETITIONS: Do fifteen. Rest for fifteen seconds, then try again. Your goal is three sets of fifteen.

Remember to do these sit-ups smoothly. Do not hold your breath while doing this exercise.

Abdomen Strengthen 1

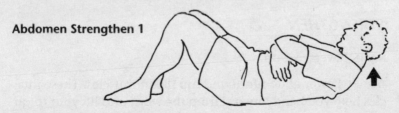

STRENGTHEN ◆ 2

NAME: 1/2 diagonal sit-up.

TARGET: External and internal abdominal obliques. These are the abdominal muscles that help you bend to the right and left.

STARTING POSITION: Lie on your back on the floor. Bend your knees so your feet are flat on the floor. Cross your arms over your chest.

THE MOTION: Slowly lift your head and chest diagonally toward one side (left shoulder toward right knee or right shoulder toward left knee).

Lift up halfway (forty-five degrees).

REPETITIONS: Do fifteen on each side. Rest for fifteen seconds. Slowly return to starting position, then try again. Your goal is three sets of fifteen.

Do them smoothly, and do not hold your breath while doing this exercise.

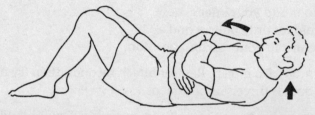

Abdomen Strengthen 2

STRENGTHEN ◆ 3

NAME: Reverse sit-up.

TARGET: Lower abdominal and hip flexor muscles. These muscles help you bend forward from the waist and lift your thigh.

STARTING POSITION: Lie on your back on the floor. Your arms should be crossed over your chest.

THE MOTION: Bend your knees so your feet are flat on the floor.

Slowly lift both knees back all the way toward your chest.

Hold for one second, then slowly return to the starting position.

REPETITIONS: Do fifteen, then rest for fifteen seconds. Then try again—your goal is three sets of fifteen.

Do them smoothly and do not hold your breath while doing this exercise.

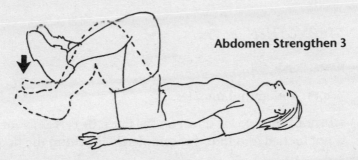

Abdomen Strengthen 3

STRENGTHEN ◆ 4

NAME: Abdominal crunch.

TARGET: All abdominal muscles.

STARTING POSITION: Lie on the floor, flat on your back. Cross your arms over your chest.

THE MOTION: Slowly lift your legs, head, and neck toward the middle of your stomach.

Hold for a count of one, then slowly return to starting position.

Abdomen Strengthen 4

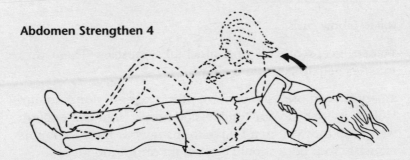

REPETITIONS: Perform two sets of fifteen. Rest fifteen seconds between each group.

Do the exercises smoothly, and remember to keep breathing throughout them.

STRENGTHEN ◆ 5

NAME: Pelvic tilt.

TARGET: Abdominal muscles.

STARTING POSITION: Lie down on the floor. Be certain your back is not arched and that it is completely touching the floor.

THE MOTION: Bend your knees so your feet are flat on the floor. Place your hands on your stomach. Tighten your stomach muscles. Be certain your lower back is in contact with the floor at all times.

REPETITIONS: Hold for five seconds. Do ten.

Do not hold your breath while doing this exercise.

Elbow

STRENGTHEN ◆ 1

NAME: Elbow curls.

TARGET: Biceps brachii and brachialis muscles. These arm muscles help to bend your elbow.

STARTING POSITION: You perform this exercise standing up. Hold a weight in your trouble side hand. Hold just enough weight so that you don't have to move your back to do this exercise. Your back should be straight and stationary.

THE MOTION: Keeping that hand at your side, palm up, bend your elbow, bringing the weighted hand up to your shoulder.
Slowly lower the hand back to your side.

REPETITIONS: Perform two sets of fifteen exercises. Rest twenty seconds after each set.

STRENGTHEN ◆ 2

NAME: Elbow extension.

TARGET: Triceps muscles. These arm muscles are used to straighten your elbow.

STARTING POSITION: Lie down on a bed or floor while holding on to a dumbbell or cuff weight.

THE MOTION: Without bending your elbow, lift the weight straight up over your body.
Then, slowly bend and straighten your elbow.

REPETITIONS: Perform two sets of fifteen. Go back to the starting position between sets and rest for twenty seconds.

Forearm

STRENGTHEN ◆ 1

NAME: Forearm pronation.

TARGET: Pronator teres and pronator quadratus muscles. These muscles are used to rotate the palm of your hand downwards.

STARTING POSITION: Place your trouble side forearm on a table in front of you. Hold on to a hammer or dumbbell weighing up to ten pounds. Your hand should be thumb side up.

THE MOTION: Slowly turn your forearm so your palm faces downward toward the table.

Hold for a count of one second.

Reverse direction to the starting position.

REPETITIONS: Perform three sets of fifteen exercises. Rest for ten seconds between sets.

Always support your elbow on a hard surface. Do not grip the hammer or dumbbell too tightly.

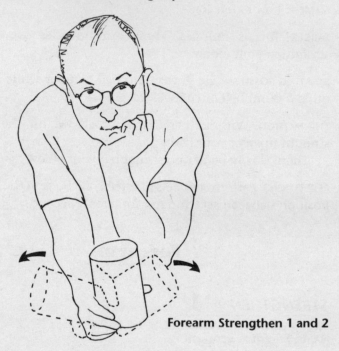

Forearm Strengthen 1 and 2

STRENGTHEN ◆ 2

NAME: Forearm supination.

TARGET: Biceps brachii and supinator muscles. These forearm muscles help to rotate the palm of your hand upward.

STARTING POSITION: Place your trouble side forearm on a table in front of you. Hold on to a hammer or dumbbell weighing up to ten pounds. Be certain your hand is thumb side up.

THE MOTION: Slowly turn your hand so that the palm faces upward.

Hold for a count of one, then return to starting position.

REPETITIONS: Perform three sets of fifteen exercises. Rest for ten seconds between sets.

Always support your elbow on a hard surface, and don't grip the hammer or dumbbell too tightly.

Wrist

STRENGTHEN ◆ 1

NAME: Wrist curl.

TARGET: Wrist flexor muscles. These muscles help bend your wrist, hand, and elbow.

STARTING POSITION: Place your forearm on the edge of a table or counter. Your wrist should be hanging off the edge, palm up. Hold a weight up to ten pounds (starting with a soup can will do) in that hand.

THE MOTION: Curl your wrist upward.

Hold for one second.

Then return to starting position.

REPETITIONS: Perform three sets of fifteen exercises. Rest ten seconds between sets.

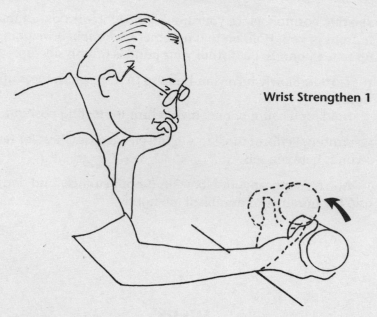

Wrist Strengthen 1

Always support your forearm on a hard surface, and do not grip the weight too tightly.

STRENGTHEN ◆ **2**

NAME: Wrist lifts.

TARGET: Wrist extensor muscles. These muscles help to lift your wrist and hand.

STARTING POSITION: Put your forearm on the edge of a table or counter. Your hand should be hanging off the edge, palm down.

THE MOTION: With a weight up to ten pounds in that hand (a soup can will do nicely), curl your wrist upward.

Hold for one second.

Then return to the starting position.

REPETITIONS: Perform three sets of ten exercises. Rest for ten seconds between sets.

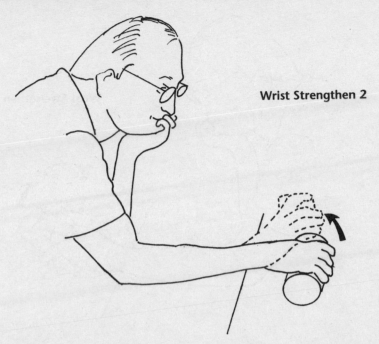

Wrist Strengthen 2

Support your forearm on a hard surface, and do not grip the weight too tightly.

STRENGTHEN ◆ 3

NAME: Wrist side pulls.

TARGET: Radial deviator muscles. These muscles help move your hand sideways in the direction of your thumb.

STARTING POSITION: Place your forearm on a table or on your lap. Turn your hand on its side with your thumb pointed upward. Hold on to a weight up to ten pounds (a hammer or a soup can is fine).

THE MOTION: Without moving your forearm, and moving only your wrist, lift the weight upward.

Hold for a count of one second.

Then slowly lower your hand to its starting position.

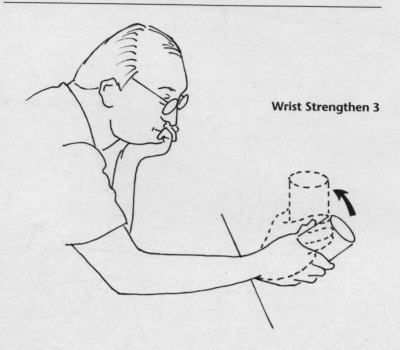

Wrist Strengthen 3

REPETITIONS: Perform three sets of fifteen. Rest for twenty seconds between sets.

Be careful not to grip the weight too tightly.

Finger

STRENGTHEN ◆ 1

NAME: Ball squeezes.

TARGET: The flexor muscles in your hand, which are responsible for bending your fingers.

STARTING POSITION: Hold a small rubber ball or a tennis ball in the palm of your hand.

THE MOTION: Keeping your wrist and forearm in a straight line, squeeze the ball tightly.

Hold each squeeze for a count of three.

Relax your grip for a count of three.

REPETITIONS: Do fifty times.

STRENGTHEN ◆ 2

NAME: Finger spreads with rubber band.

TARGET: The extensor muscles in your hand, which are responsible for straightening all of your fingers.

STARTING POSITION: Find a rubber band that can fit around your fingers, including your thumb. Keep your wrist and forearm in a straight line.

THE MOTION: Slowly spread your fingers apart against the tension of the rubber band.

Hold for a count of one.

Relax your hand for a count of one.

REPETITIONS: Do it fifty times, rest for thirty seconds. Repeat the process once more.

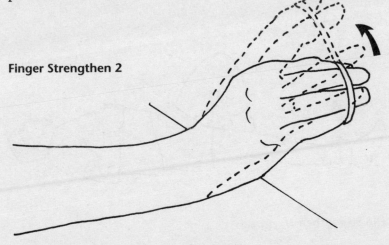

Finger Strengthen 2

Hip

STRENGTHEN ◆ 1

NAME: Straight leg raise.

TARGET: The quadriceps, which help to bring your thigh forward and straighten your leg.

STARTING POSITION: Place a weight around the ankle of the leg you want to strengthen. Lie down on your back, and bend your other leg. This will help protect your back. Keep the trouble side leg straight.

THE MOTION: Lift the leg—weight and all. It's crucial that you *do not bend this knee.*

Lift your leg to the height of the knee that is bent—there's no need to go any higher than that.

Increase the weight so that eventually it matches 10 percent of your total body weight. If you weigh 120 pounds, for example, your goal should be 12 pounds.

REPETITIONS: Perform two sets of ten leg lifts. Rest twenty seconds between sets.

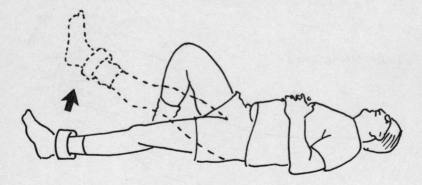

Hip Strengthen 1

STRENGTHEN ◆ 2

NAME: Straight leg raise with foot rotated outward.

TARGET: Vastus medialis oblique muscle, which helps to straighten your leg.

STARTING POSITION: Place a weight around the trouble side ankle or foot. Lie down on your back, and bend your other leg. This will help protect your back.

THE MOTION: Rotate the injured leg so that your foot is pointing outward. *Do not bend the knee of this leg.*

Lift to the height of the knee that is bent.

Increase the weight gradually with a goal of 10 percent of your total body weight.

REPETITIONS: Perform two sets of ten leg lifts. Rest twenty seconds between sets.

STRENGTHEN ◆ 3

NAME: Hip side lifts.

TARGET: Gluteus medius and tensor fasciae latae muscles, which help move your leg out to the side.

STARTING POSITION: Place a weight around the trouble side ankle or foot. Lie on your side with the leg/hip to be exercised on top. Bend the bottom leg for support. *Do not bend the top leg!*

THE MOTION: Lift your top leg upward until it forms a straight line with the rest of your body.

Then lower the leg slowly.

The goal of the weight to be lifted should be 10 percent of your total body weight.

REPETITIONS: Perform two sets of ten exercises. Rest for twenty seconds between sets.

STRENGTHEN ◆ 4

NAME: Inner thigh lifts.

TARGET: Groin muscles, which help you squeeze your legs together.

STARTING POSITION: Place a weight around your trouble side ankle or foot. Lie on your side with the leg/hip to be exercised on the bottom. Cross your top leg over your bottom leg.

THE MOTION: Lift your bottom leg six inches off the surface you're lying on. *Do not bend that knee.*
  The goal of the weight to be lifted should be 10 percent of your total body weight.

REPETITIONS: Perform two sets of ten lifts. Rest for twenty seconds between sets.

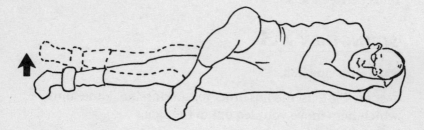

Hip Strengthen 4

STRENGTHEN ◆ 5

NAME: Hip flexion.

TARGET: Iliopsoas muscles. These two muscles located in the front of your hip help lift your thigh.

STARTING POSITION: Place a weight around your trouble side ankle or foot. Sit up on a high stool or on the edge of a table or bed.

THE MOTION: While keeping your back straight, place your hands at your side.

Lift up the knee on the side to be exercised six inches.

The weight placed on your foot or ankle should eventually reach 10 percent of your total body weight.

REPETITIONS: Perform two sets of ten exercises. Rest twenty seconds between sets.

Don't lean too far back or forward during this exercise. Keep your back as straight as possible.

Knee

STRENGTHEN ◆ 1

NAME: Leg curls.

TARGET: Hamstrings. Located in the back of your thigh, these muscles help move your leg backward and bend your knee.

STARTING POSITION: This exercise is performed while standing. Place a weight around your ankle.

THE MOTION: With your hands in front of you, hold on to a table or back of a chair for support.

Bend the trouble side knee and bring the weighted foot up toward your butt.

Halfway up is sufficient.

Eventually, your goal should be to use a weight equal to 10 percent of your total body weight.

REPETITIONS: Perform two sets of ten exercises. Rest twenty seconds between sets.

Try not to lean forward while performing this exercise.

STRENGTHEN ◆ 2

NAME: Mini squats.

TARGET: The quadriceps help move your thigh forward and straighten your leg.

STARTING POSITION: Stand straight up and spread your legs about twelve inches apart.

THE MOTION: With your hands on hips, bend your knees about one-quarter of a full squat.

Then return to a standing position.

When you're comfortable doing this, you might want to place weights in each hand, as heavy as you can handle without a strain or struggle.

REPETITIONS: Perform three sets of twenty squats. Rest twenty seconds between sets.

If you feel *any* knee pain, discontinue this exercise immediately. Never bend your knees more than one-quarter of a full squat. Otherwise you may create new pain.

STRENGTHEN ◆ 3

NAME: Terminal knee extension.

TARGET: Quadriceps muscles.

STARTING POSITION: You can sit up or lie down for this exercise.

THE MOTION: Roll up two or three towels together, making a cylinder out of them.

Put the towel roll under the knee on your trouble side.

Straighten the knee by lifting your leg. You should be lifting only your leg, not your thigh.

Knee Strengthen 3

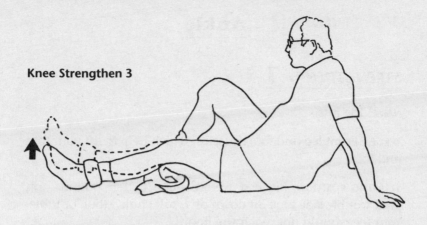

REPETITIONS: Perform two sets of fifteen exercises. Rest twenty seconds between sets.

Adding a weight to your ankle is desirable if you can handle it. Do not use more than 10 percent of your total body weight. If you feel any knee pain, discontinue this exercise immediately.

STRENGTHEN ◆ 4

NAME: Quad sets.

TARGET: Quadriceps.

STARTING POSITION: Sit up or lie down on any flat surface with both legs straight out in front of you.

THE MOTION: Tighten the thigh muscle of the injured leg while trying to press the back of your knee flat against the surface.
Hold for a count of six.
Then rest for a count of one.

REPETITIONS: Do twenty of these exercises.

Ankle

STRENGTHEN ◆ 1

NAME: Toe lifts.

TARGET: Front leg and foot muscles, which help to lift your foot and toes.

STARTING POSITION: Place a weight—five to ten pounds—on your trouble side foot. Sit down on a tall chair, stool, or table. Your feet should not reach the floor.

THE MOTION: Point your weighted foot so that the toe is up, without lifting your thigh.

REPETITIONS: Perform three sets of fifteen exercises. Rest twenty seconds between sets.

STRENGTHEN ◆ 2

NAME: Heel lifts.

TARGET: Gastrocnemius soleus muscles, which help you move up on your toes when walking, running, and jumping.

STARTING POSITION: Stand on a step, curb, or even a pile of books—phone books work best—and put your hands in front of you. Hold on to the back of a chair or a wall for support while letting your heels hang off the edge of the books.

THE MOTION: Slowly lift yourself up on the balls of your feet. When you're strong enough, try it one foot at a time.

REPETITIONS: Perform two sets of twenty exercises each. Rest for twenty seconds between sets.

STRENGTHEN ◆ 3

NAME: Ankle inversion.

TARGET: Tibialis anterior and posterior muscles. These are used to turn your foot inward.

STARTING POSITION: Lie on your side on a hard surface. A table or a bench is fine. Your trouble side foot should be on the bottom, closest to the hard surface. Place a weight on the trouble side foot and let that foot hang off the edge.

THE MOTION: Slowly lift the weighted foot upward. The inside of your foot should be facing the ceiling.

It may be more comfortable if you place a towel on the surface for the weighted foot to rest on between lifts.

REPETITIONS: Perform two sets of fifteen exercises each. Work toward lifting a ten-pound weight.

STRENGTHEN ◆ 4

NAME: Ankle eversion.

TARGET: Peroneus longus and brevis muscles. These help move your foot outward.

STARTING POSITION: Lie on a hard surface such as a table or bench. The foot you want to strengthen should be on top. Place a weight on that foot and let it hang off the edge.

THE MOTION: You'll have to bend your bottom leg to make this work.

Slowly lift your weighted foot toward the ceiling. As you do, the outside of your ankle should be facing upward.

It may be more comfortable if you place a towel on the surface when you rest your ankle between lifts.

REPETITIONS: Perform three sets of fifteen exercises. Rest twenty seconds between sets.

Work toward lifting a ten-pound weight.

Foot

STRENGTHEN ◆ 1

NAME: Towel crunches.

TARGET: Sole of foot.

STARTING POSITION: Place a towel on the floor. Sit on a chair and place your troubled foot on the towel.

THE MOTION: Try to "scrunch" up or wrinkle the towel by moving your toes and arching your foot.

REPETITIONS: Perform two sets of fifty crunches. Rest for fifteen seconds between sets.

Towel Crunch

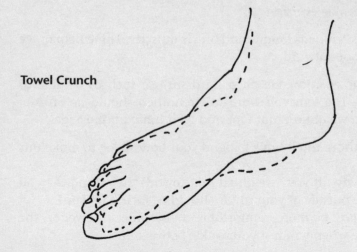

BALANCE ◆ 1

Stand on one leg for sixty seconds. It's okay to hold on to something to maintain your balance.

Rest for ten seconds.

Do a repeat performance, but this time with your eyes closed.

Do these exercises in sets of five.

BALANCE ◆ 2

Standing on one leg, then the other, play catch with yourself.

Toss the ball in the air or against a wall a total of twenty times.

Rest for ten seconds.

Repeat the process five times.

BALANCE ◆ 3

Hop in place on one leg.

Then the other.

Do a total of thirty hops, then pause ten seconds.

Repeat the process five times.

GLOSSARY

Acute We use this term to refer to intense pain. It is also used to describe an injury that has recently occurred or symptoms of which have come on quickly.

Arthritis The wearing away of the cartilage surface in any joint of the body. This is accompanied by pain, swelling, and stiffness.

Biomechanics The interaction of your muscles and bones when you call on them to perform a task.

Bone Made primarily of calcium and phosphorus, it provides shape and support to the body. It also serves as an attachment site for muscles and ligaments.

Brace Made of various materials, it is used to support weak or injured parts of the body.

Bursa This fluid-filled sac contains synovial fluid. There are many of them throughout your body, located near the joints or other areas with irregular surfaces. Its purpose is to reduce friction between tendons and a bone.

Bursitis The condition when the bursa becomes inflamed, filling with more synovial fluid, causing pain and discomfort.

Charley horse The pain and tenderness that comes from damage to muscle fibers. It could be the result of a muscle strain, tear, or contusion.

Chronic Any problem that doesn't change much, but lingers on.

Contraction A tightening of a muscle in order to cause a movement.

Contracture A permanent shortening of a muscle.

Contusion A muscle bruise.

Electrolytes   The concentration of sodium, potassium, and chloride found in some body fluids, which provides the basis for nerve functions.

Fibrosis   An excessive formation of scar tissue in a muscle or joint.

Flexibility   How far you can move, and the ease with which you do it.

Gait   The way you walk.

Inflammation   An increase in blood flow that causes swelling in and around an injury.

Joint   The area where two bones meet, aiding in their movement.

Joint capsule   The covering of two bones at the area where they meet. It helps support the joint and provides it with essential nutrients.

Ligament   The fibrous collagen tissue connecting a bone to a bone. It provides stability to a joint.

Muscle   A fibrous structure that tightens, creates tension, and pulls on your bones to create movement.

Nerve   The electric wiring of your body. Nerves are responsible for sensing things and turning muscles on and off.

Paratenon   A fibrous covering of a tendon.

Periosteum   A fibrous membrane that covers your bones.

Pronation   Poor alignment of the foot and ankle that is one of the causes of flat feet.

Range of motion   How far you can move your arms, legs, and other joints.

Spasm   The sudden and involuntary contraction of a muscle.

Sprain/Strain   A tearing of muscle or ligament fibers.

Sterile   Something that is germ free.

Strength   How much force you can produce through your muscles.

Stretch   Increasing the flexibility of a muscle or a joint.

Supination   A poor alignment of the foot and ankle, which is one of the causes of high arches.

Syndrome   A set of various symptoms that describe a disease or abnormal condition.

Tendinitis   Inflammation of the tendons.

Tendon   The tissue that connects muscle to bone, aiding in the bone's movement.

◆ ABOUT THE AUTHORS ◆

Morton Dean
and
Benjamin Gelfand, P.T.

This book is the product of aches and pains and the dreams of our Glory Days. Veteran TV news correspondent Morton Dean comes to the project as an award-winning news correspondent and long-suffering jock.

For over forty years he has covered many of the world's most historic news events. Dean is not content to sit back and be a spectator of our changing world. And he's not content to be a sports spectator, either. For years he has struggled—successfully, he believes—to remain in good physical condition and retain his competitive edge. It has not been a pain-free quest.

A spectacular record of aches and pains validates his dedication. In part, it's been a lifelong attempt to overcome a gnawing, psychological impairment brought about by spending too much time on the bench as a high school athlete. However, in his lengthy resume, Mort prefers to emphasize the fact that he did play—and charm—his way into the captaincy of the Emerson College basketball team, in Boston. It was not a Final Four kind of atmosphere, but it was a team nevertheless. And it can be certified that he was the captain. It was there that he honed his skills as an overachiever.

Aging witnesses testify that Mort appears to have triumphed over time and that he is a more versatile and more skilled athlete now. He does not dispute that analysis. He is a jogger, tennis player, skier, sailor, and softball player.

It was at his weekly softball game that he realized the need for an easy reference guide to the injuries suffered by aging, part-time jocks. Every Sunday Mort and his summertime Glory Days teammates, suffering from a variety of physically enervating, ego-damaging pulls and sprains, held repetitive conversations about what advice to follow.

Do you ice it? Is heat the best treatment? Get off it? Or play through the pain? Stretch it out? Or pack it in? See you in one

253

week? Or will it take three or four? What kind of rehab is necessary? Clearly, a book that had answers to all those questions and tells the aging jock specifically what kind of first aid he should give himself and how he can limit and possibly prevent future risk was needed.

Mort's frequent muscle pulls brought him to the famous Nicholas Institute of Sports Medicine run by a pioneer in the field, the revered Dr. James Nicholas. It was there, while rehabbing an aching leg, that Mort and another Glory Days jock, Ben Gelfand, teamed up to work on this book.

For years, Ben had been dealing with his own aches and pains. And especially those of others! He's the supervisor of the Nicholas Institute and taught at NYU, where he received his degree in physical therapy. Ben's real Glory Days began in the eighth grade when he first made his mark as a competitive runner.

He fulfilled the promise of stardom as captain and MVP of his high school track team. Later, he lettered in track at the State University of New York at Stony Brook and also at New York University. An old advertisement testifies to Ben's superlative performances. In full gallop he's featured in a promotion for the famed Penn Relays. It's his favorite poster. Not content to live off the vicarious thrills of his physically active patients, Ben continues to run competitively and expand his reach to include marathons.